Diagnostic Pathology

Editor

VICKIE L. COOPER

VETERINARY CLINICS OF NORTH AMERICA: FOOD ANIMAL PRACTICE

www.vetfood.theclinics.com

Consulting Editor
ROBERT A. SMITH

November 2012 • Volume 28 • Number 3

ELSEVIER

1600 John F. Kennedy Boulevard • Suite 1800 • Philadelphia, PA 19103-2899

http://www.vetfood.theclinics.com

VETERINARY CLINICS OF NORTH AMERICA: FOOD ANIMAL PRACTICE Volume 28, Number 3
November 2012 ISSN 0749-0720, ISBN-13: 978-1-4557-4969-0

Editor: John Vassallo; j.vassallo@elsevier.com
Developmental Editor: Teia Stone

Veterinary Clinics of North America: Food Animal Practice (ISSN 0749-0720) is published in March, July, and November by Elsevier Inc., 360 Park Avenue South, New York, NY 10010-1710. Subscription prices are $215.00 per year (domestic individuals), $296.00 per year (domestic institutions), $100.00 per year (domestic students/residents), $243.00 per year (Canadian individuals), $387.00 per year (Canadian institutions), $307.00 per year (international individuals), $387.00 per year (international institutions), and $153.00 per year (international and Canadian students/residents). To receive student/resident rate, orders must be accompanied by name of affiliated institution, date of term, and the signature of program/residency coordinator on institution letterhead. *Clinics* subscription prices. All prices are subject to change without notice. **POSTMASTER:** Send address changes to *Veterinary Clinics of North America: Food Animal Practice*, Elsevier Health Sciences Division, Subscription Customer Service, 3251 Riverport Lane, Maryland Heights, MO 63043. Customer Service (orders, claims, online, change of address): Elsevier Health Sciences Division, Subscription Customer Service, 3251 Riverport Lane, Maryland Heights, MO 63043. Tel: 1-800-654-2452 (U.S. and Canada); 314-447-8871 (ouside U.S. and Canada). Fax: 314-447-8029. E-mail: journalscustomerservice-usa@elsevier.com (for print support); journalsonlinesupport-usa@elsevier.com (for online support).

Reprints. For copies of 100 or more, of articles in this publication, please contact the Commercial Reprints Department, Elsevier Inc., 360 Park Avenue South, New York, NY 10010-1710. Tel.: 212-633-3812; Fax: 212-462-1935; E-mail: reprints@elsevier.com.

Veterinary Clinics of North America: Food Animal Practice is covered in *Current Contents/Agriculture, Biology and Environmental Sciences, MEDLINE/PubMed (Index Medicus), and Excerpta Medica.*

Printed and bound by CPI Group (UK) Ltd, Croydon, CR0 4YY

Transferred to digital print 2012

Contributors

CONSULTING EDITOR

ROBERT A. SMITH, DVM, MS
Diplomate, American Board of Veterinary Practitioners; Veterinary Research and
Consulting Services, LLC, Greeley, Colorado

GUEST EDITOR

VICKIE L. COOPER, DVM, MS, PhD
Senior Clinician, Department of Veterinary Diagnostic and Production Animal Medicine,
College of Veterinary Medicine, Iowa State University, Ames, Iowa

AUTHORS

KEN BATEMAN, DVM, MSc
Associate Professor, Department of Population Medicine, Ontario Veterinary College,
University of Guelph, Guelph, Ontario, Canada

ROBERT J. BILDFELL, DVM, MSc
Associate Professor, Department of Biomedical Sciences, College of Veterinary Medicine,
Oregon State University, Corvallis, Oregon

PATRICIA CAREY BLANCHARD, DVM, PhD
Diagnostic Pathologist and Tulare Branch Chief, University of California Animal Health and
Food Safety Laboratory, School of Veterinary Medicine, University of California-Davis,
Tulare, California

BRUCE W. BRODERSEN, DVM, MS, PhD
Assistant Professor, Veterinary Diagnostic Center, School of Veterinary Medicine and
Biomedical Sciences, University of Nebraska-Lincoln, Lincoln, Nebraska

JEFF L. CASWELL, DVM, DVSc, PhD
Diplomate, American College of Veterinary Pathologists; Professor, Department of
Pathobiology, Ontario Veterinary College, University of Guelph, Guelph, Ontario, Canada

EDWARD G. CLARK, DVM, MVSc
Diplomate, American College of Veterinary Pathologists; Calgary, Alberta, Canada

JOSEPHA DELAY, DVM, DVSc
Diplomate, American College of Veterinary Pathologists; Animal Health Laboratory,
University of Guelph, Ontario, Canada

STEVE ENSLEY, DVM, PhD
Senior Clinician, Veterinary Diagnostic Laboratory, College of Veterinary Medicine, Iowa
State University, Ames, Iowa

GLORIA GIOIA, PhD
Quality Milk Production Services, College of Veterinary Medicine, Cornell University, Ithaca, New York; Department of Veterinary Science and Public Health, Università degli Studi di Milano, Milan, Italy

DEE GRIFFIN, DVM, MS
Beef Cattle Production Management Veterinarian, Great Plains Veterinary Educational Center, Clay Center, Nebraska

ABHIJIT GURJAR, DVM, PhD
Quality Milk Production Services, College of Veterinary Medicine, Cornell University, Ithaca, New York

JOANNE HEWSON, DVM, PhD
Diplomate, American College of Veterinary Internal Medicine (Large Animal); Associate Professor, Department of Clinical Studies, Ontario Veterinary College, University of Guelph, Guelph, Ontario, Canada

LARRY D. HOLLER, DVM, PhD
Reproductive Disease Specialist, Animal Disease Research and Diagnostic Laboratory, Professor, Veterinary and Biomedical Sciences Department, South Dakota State University, Brookings, South Dakota

CHRISTIANE V. LÖHR, Dr Med Vet, PhD
Associate Professor, Department of Biomedical Sciences, College of Veterinary Medicine, Oregon State University, Corvallis, Oregon

CATHERINE G. LAMM, DVM, MRCVS
Diplomate, American College of Veterinary Pathologists; Lecturer, School of Veterinary Medicine, University of Glasgow, Bearsden, Glasgow, United Kingdom

PAOLO MORONI, DVM, PhD
Quality Milk Production Services, College of Veterinary Medicine, Cornell University, Ithaca, New York; Department of Health, Animal Science and Food Safety, Università degli Studi di Milano, Milan, Italy

JEROME C. NIETFELD, DVM, PhD
Diplomate, American College of Veterinary Pathologists; Professor, Department of Diagnostic Medicine/Pathobiology, College of Veterinary Medicine, Kansas State University, Manhattan, Kansas

BRADLEY L. NJAA, DVM, MVSc
Diplomate, American College of Veterinary Pathologists; Associate Professor, Department of Pathobiology, Center for Veterinary Health Sciences, Oklahoma State University, Stillwater, Oklahoma

ROGER J. PANCIERA, DVM, PhD
Diplomate, American College of Veterinary Pathologists; Professor Emeritus, Department of Pathobiology, Center for Veterinary Health Sciences, Oklahoma State University, Stillwater, Oklahoma

WILSON RUMBEIHA, DVM, PhD
Diplomate, American Board of Toxicology; Diplomate, American Board of Veterinary Toxicology; Professor, Veterinary Diagnostic Laboratory, College of Veterinary Medicine, Iowa State University, Ames, Iowa

YNTE SCHUKKEN, DVM, PhD
Quality Milk Production Services, College of Veterinary Medicine, Cornell University, Ithaca, New York

JAN K. SHEARER, DVM, MS
Professor and Dairy Extension Specialist, Veterinary Diagnostic and Production Animal Medicine, College of Veterinary Medicine, Iowa State University, Ames, Iowa

ĐURĐA SLAVIĆ, DVM, MSc, PhD
Animal Health Laboratory, University of Guelph, Ontario, Canada

DAVID R. SMITH, DVM, PhD
Diplomate, Epidemiology Specialty American College of Veterinary Preventive Medicine, Department of Pathobiology and Population Medicine, College of Veterinary Medicine, Mississippi

SUSAN J. TORNQUIST, DVM, PhD
Professor, Department of Biomedical Sciences, College of Veterinary Medicine, Oregon State University, Corvallis, Oregon

SAREL R. VAN AMSTEL, BVSc, Dip Med Vet, M MED VET
Diplomate, American College of Veterinary Internal Medicine; Professor, Department of Large Animal Clinical Sciences, College of Veterinary Medicine, The University of Tennessee, Knoxville, Tennessee

FRANK WELCOME, DVM, MBA
Quality Milk Production Services, College of Veterinary Medicine, Cornell University, Ithaca, New York

RUTH ZADOKS, DVM, PhD
Quality Milk Production Services, College of Veterinary Medicine, Cornell University, Ithaca, New York; Moredun Research Institute, Pentlands Science Park, Penicuik, Midlothian, Scotland

Contents

> Field necropsies can provide a wealth of information that can help guide production management decisions. Techniques outlined can allow a veterinary practitioner to complete a thorough necropsy of a bovine, including examination of the brain when indicated, in less than 20 minutes. An observation and history collection system using form templates and photographs is outlined that improves efficiency of recording necropsy results. One key to necropsy efficiency, speed, and enjoyment is having sharp knives. The first part of the article includes tips for sharpening knives. The article also includes detailed information on appropriate diagnostic specimen handling, packaging, and shipping.

> Successful abortion diagnosis in ruminants involves input from the producer, practitioner, and diagnostician. Unfortunately, despite best efforts, many investigations still result in a diagnosis of idiopathic abortion. If this diagnosis is made after a complete and systematic investigation of appropriate and reasonably preserved samples, some comfort can be taken that practitioners and diagnosticians did their best for the benefit of the producer. As new diagnostic technology is developed for abortion diseases, hopefully this best will only get better.

> Pathologic and laboratory investigations are essential when identification of the specific cause of bovine respiratory disease is needed. Considerations for planning a diagnostic investigation include the goals of the inquiry, the potential impact of the diagnosis, the plausible causes based on the clinical and epidemiologic appearance, and the relative merits of the available diagnostic strategies. This review uses 4 cases to outline different approaches to laboratory diagnosis. The postmortem examination is described, along with the patterns and gross appearance of lesions, considerations for effective sampling from appropriately selected animals, and reasons for discrepant or negative laboratory test results.

> Calf diarrhea is a multifactorial disease related to a combination of host and pathogen factors. The most common pathogens found in diarrheic

calves are cryptosporidium, rotavirus, coronavirus, *Salmonella,* attaching and effacing *E coli* and F5 (K99) *Escherichia coli.* Increased mortality and morbidity are often due to the presence of more than one pathogen. This article includes a discussion of key information to obtain a clinical history, the pathogens, pathology findings, and diagnostic methods.

Diarrhea is a leading cause of sickness and death of beef and dairy calves in their first month of life. Field investigations of outbreaks of neonatal calf diarrhea should be conducted for the purposes of (1) reducing the losses associated with existing cases and (2) preventing new cases from occurring. The appropriate corrective actions are determined by taking a population approach to diagnostics and prevention. It can be difficult to provide solutions to disease outbreaks, but success is more likely if an organized, epidemiologic approach to outbreak investigation is followed.

The purpose of the gross necropsy examination of the gastrointestinal tract is to recognize the presence of lesions, thus requiring a basic understanding of its normal appearance and anatomy. This article highlights gross changes to the gastrointestinal tract of adult cattle that help place the disease processes into broad categories. Although few gross lesions reach the zenith of pathognomonic, there are numerous lesions that, when considered in aggregate with history (eg, number of animals affected, environment, duration of signs, time of onset relative to management changes, previous management) and clinical signs, can help narrow the spectrum of causes, provide a basis for a strong presumptive diagnosis, and focus diagnostic test selection.

Diseases of the central nervous system (CNS) are relatively common in food animals. Potential causes include infectious agents, nutritional deficiencies, metabolic disorders, genetic defects, toxins, and idiopathic causes. Determining the correct etiologic diagnosis often depends on a thorough postmortem examination and collection of samples. This article reviews some of the steps and procedures necessary to collect the necessary information on CNS diseases in food animals. Techniques for the examination of the CNS are briefly described, and some of the gross pathology likely to be encountered in a food animal practice is reviewed.

The causes of lameness in cattle are multifactorial and involve a combination of housing, management, and environmental factors and a variety of infectious agents. Arriving at a cause can often require concerted efforts.

Diagnosis of lameness is often based mainly on clinical observations. A detailed record of those observations with time and among several animals within a herd can provide valuable information toward solving lameness problems. Advances in computer hardware and software help facilitate more detailed data collection and analysis.

VETERINARY CLINICS OF NORTH AMERICA: FOOD ANIMAL PRACTICE

FORTHCOMING ISSUES

March 2013
Pain Management
Hans Coetzee, BVSc, PhD, MRCVS,
Guest Editor

July 2013
Metabolic Diseases of Ruminants
Thomas H. Herdt, DVM, MS, *Guest Editor*

RECENT ISSUES

July 2012
Mastitis in Dairy Cows
Pamela L. Ruegg, DVM, MPVM,
Guest Editor

March 2012
Evidence-Based Veterinary Medicine for the Bovine Veterinarian
Sébastien Buczinski, Dr Vét, DÉS, MSc,
and Jean-Michel Vandeweerd, DMV, MS,
Guest Editors

November 2011
Johne's Disease
Michael T. Collins, DVM, PhD,
Guest Editor

RELATED INTEREST

Veterinary Clinics of North America: Equine Practice
April 2012 (Vol. 28, No. 1)
Ambulatory Practice
David W. Ramey, DVM, and Mark R. Baus, DVM, *Guest Editors*

THE CLINICS ARE NOW AVAILABLE ONLINE!
Access your subscription at:
www.theclinics.com

Preface

Diagnostic Pathology

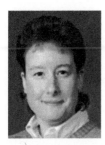

Vickie L. Cooper, DVM, MS, PhD
Guest Editor

When agreeing to be guest editor of this issue of *Veterinary Clinics of North America: Food Animal Practice*, my goal was to not only present current information related to pathology and diagnostics but also provide a quick source of reminders. Every effort has been made to keep this issue practical and useful, while providing sound science.

I would like to extend my appreciation for contributions from all the authors. This is a group of diagnosticians, pathologists, toxicologists, epidemiologists, and practicing veterinarians that have been a pleasure with which to work. I would also like to thank John Vassallo, Editor, at the Saunders/Elsevier Company for his patience and guidance with this issue. I would like to thank Dr Bob Smith for his encouragement. Last, but certainly not least, many thanks to my husband for his support.

Vickie L. Cooper, DVM, MS, PhD
Department of Veterinary Diagnostic and Production Animal Medicine
College of Veterinary Medicine, Iowa State University
1600 South 16th Street
Ames, IA 50011, USA

E-mail address:
vcooper@iastate.edu

Vet Clin Food Anim 28 (2012) xi
http://dx.doi.org/10.1016/j.cvfa.2012.07.012
0749-0720/12/$ – see front matter
vetfood.theclinics.com

Field Necropsy of Cattle and Diagnostic Sample Submission

Dee Griffin, DVM, MS

KEYWORDS

- Bovine • Necropsy • Diagnostic • Sharpening knives • Shipping specimens
- Data collection

KEY POINTS

- Field necropsies can provide a wealth of information that can help guide production management decisions.
- The outlined procedures emphasize not detaching organs from the carcass unless necessary, thereby making carcass removal by rendering companies more efficient and minimizing clean-up on the production unit premise.
- An observation and history collection system using form templates and photographs improves efficiency of recording necropsy results.
- One key to necropsy efficiency, speed, and enjoyment is having sharp knives. The first part of the article includes tips for sharpening knives.

FIELD NECROPSY AND DIAGNOSTIC SAMPLE SUBMISSION

This section includes:

- A brief overview of knife-sharpening skills and sharpening tools
- A step-by-step field necropsy technique for ruminants
- Review of simplified observations collection
- Techniques for handling laboratory samples including proper packaging and shipping of samples to diagnostic facilities

The principal purpose of field necropsies is to gain information that may be used to evaluate production or influence production management decisions. Many production management issues relate to making a complete and thorough assessment of organ systems, including their associated lymph nodes.

Safety is paramount, so always have protective clothing, gloves, and boots that allow for disinfection. Remind all bystanders and observers of the importance of being careful to minimize their personal contamination. Have water, soap, disinfectant, and cleaning brushes readily available.

The author has no disclosures as part of the complete article.
Great Plains Veterinary Educational Center, Highway 18 Spur, PO Box 148, Clay Center, NE 68933-0148, USA
E-mail address: dgriffin@gpvec.unl.edu

Vet Clin Food Anim 28 (2012) 391–405
http://dx.doi.org/10.1016/j.cvfa.2012.07.006
0749-0720/12/$ – see front matter

KNIFE-SHARPENING SKILLS

A quick alternative to using a knife-sharpening abrasive is to use a "V" carbide blade knife sharpener. These put a very coarse, crudely shaped, yet usable edge on a knife blade.

Sharpening Abrasives

Although 3-sided oil stones work well, these are generally expensive and do not travel well when needed for field necropsies. Solid abrasives such as diamond-coated steel slabs are more durable than stone abrasives. They are easily cleaned and come in an assortment of grits. Most knives can be sharpened nicely with any abrasive that is finer than 300 grit (medium or fine).

Angle consistency, or the angle at which the blade is held as the abrasive is stroked, is by far the most important key to developing a sharp cutting edge. There are several diamond-coated sharpening abrasives designed to maintain a consistent sharpening angle. Most feature a clamp to hold the knife blade, and the abrasive is connected to a rod that slides through angle slots above and below the knife's cutting edge.

A consistent edge can be maintained on a flat abrasive if the back of the knife blade is pushed into the palm side of the thumb and the side of the thumb is laid flat against the abrasive as it is stroked (**Fig. 1**). It is difficult to maintain a consistent angle when using a diamond-coated sharpening rod or steel, and for this reason, these sharpening tools are not recommended.

The best knife-sharpening abrasives for veterinary practitioners are motorized. The author strongly encourages having a high-quality diamond-coated, set-angle disk sharpener in clinics. The better diamond hone machines have 3 sharpening stages, meaning that there are 3 slightly different angles for the abrasives. The final stage in these usually is 5° wider, which provides increased durability to the cutting edge. Diamond honing knife sharpeners can be found at most large department stores in the kitchen appliance area. Buy lots of knives and keep several sharp knives in the practice vehicle. Purchase a good-quality motorized knife sharpener and delegate the sharping to a technician.

Angles of a Sharp Cutting Edge

There is no perfect angle for a cutting edge ... but, instead, knives with a cutting edge angle not suitable for the intended job. The steeper the angle, the thinner is the blade near the cutting edge and the less durable is the cutting edge. Although durability is lost with steeper angles, the resistance caused by the knife sliding through the tissue is less. Examples include slicing knives. Similarly, the flatter the sharpening angle, the thicker is the steel to support the cutting edge and therefore the more durable. The kind of angle targeted for axes and shears is shown (**Fig. 2**). A flat file works well for

Consistent Angle Is Key to Sharpening

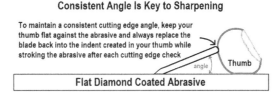

To maintain a consistent cutting edge angle, keep your thumb flat against the abrasive and always replace the blade back into the indent created in your thumb while stroking the abrasive after each cutting edge check

angle   Thumb

Flat Diamond Coated Abrasive

Fig. 1. A consistent angle can be maintained while developing a cutting edge by holding the back of the knife blade against the thumb and resting the thumb on the flat sharpening abrasive.

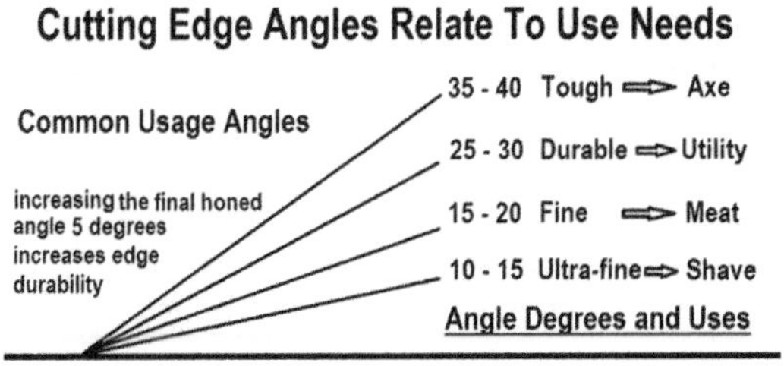

Cutting Edge Angles Relate To Use Needs

Common Usage Angles

increasing the final honed
angle 5 degrees
increases edge
durability

35 - 40 Tough ➡ Axe

25 - 30 Durable ➡ Utility

15 - 20 Fine ➡ Meat

10 - 15 Ultra-fine➡ Shave

<u>Angle Degrees and Uses</u>

Fig. 2. The angle of the knife's cutting edge determines its durability and the ease with which a sharp cutting edge slides through tissues. Select the edge best suited for the job.

sharpening the soft metal found in axes and shears. Necropsy knives seem to work well if the angle is 15° to 25°. Again, the key is keeping the angle constant when developing a cutting edge.

Finishing the Cutting Edge

A ceramic sharpening rod is one of the betters tools for honing a fine edge on a properly sharpened knife blade. When using a ceramic rod or metal steel, stroke the blade gently, feeling for defects in the cutting edge as the blade slides down the tool.

Determining When the Edge is Sharp

A sharp cutting edge should be as smooth as glass. The best and safest way to test the edge is to hold a plastic ink pen at a 45° angle and see if the knife blade will sit on the pen without sliding down the pen barrel. If it holds onto the plastic barrel, the cutting edge is sharp. Additionally, no defects should be felt when the plastic barrel of the ink pen is lightly slid down the cutting edge (**Fig. 3**).

The Keys to Having Sharp Necropsy Knives

Do not use the necropsy knife for jobs that will damage its cutting edge. For example, use a disposable bladed box cutter for skin incisions, thereby not damaging the cutting edge of the necropsy knife on hide, hair, and dirt. Do not use a necropsy knife for cutting rib cartilage unless it is of a very young animal. A shear or axe works well

TESTING THE CUTTING EDGE

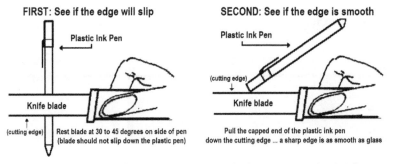

FIRST: See if the edge will slip

Plastic Ink Pen

Knife blade

(cutting edge)   Rest blade at 30 to 45 degrees on side of pen
(blade should not slip down the plastic pen)

SECOND: See if the edge is smooth

Plastic Ink Pen

(cutting edge)

Knife blade

Pull the capped end of the plastic ink pen
down the cutting edge ... a sharp edge is as smooth as glass

Fig. 3. Testing the sharpness of a cutting edge is easily done using a plastic ink pen or the thumbnail. Sharp cutting edges will grab the barrel or the thumbnail when held at a 45° angle and not slip down. Additionally, a sharp cutting edge will feel smooth as a plastic pen or thumbnail is slid down the edge.

and saves the cutting edge of the knife. Use a ceramic rod to repeatedly touch up the cutting edge during the necropsy.

FIELD NECROPSY PROCEDURE WITH MINIMAL LOOSE PARTS
Important Note

Animals that will be rendered must not contain chemical residues that could be harmful to other animals that would consume rendered products.[1]

Start with the Ruminant on its Left Side

Think about what is observed. Collect histopathologic and culture specimens while working. Histopathologic specimens should not be thicker than 5 to 7 mm. Try to connect observations into a unifying diagnosis or production management observation.

The procedure outlined is designed to make it easier for animals to be picked up by rendering trucks and to minimize hide damage, thereby improving the hide value to renderers. Detaching any organs that are not required for examination is not being considerate of the people working for the rendering company and is more likely to create a mess at the farm, ranch, or feedlot on which the necropsy examination is being performed.

Review Anatomy and Gross Pathology

Knowledge of the structure and function of the organ tissues being examined can be key to linking observations to a meaningful diagnosis.[2,3] Be slow to jump to diagnostic conclusion based on the first observations. The "lift a leg and look" or "peek-a-boo" necropsies generally leave important production management observation undiscovered and minimize the value of the observations that could have contributed to better animal care and management.

Accessing the Brain

It is important to check with the rendering company serving the animal facility about the acceptability of examining the brain, because some companies will not pick up carcasses that have had the cranium opened. Also remember that rabies should be on the differential list for all central nervous system cases, so take all appropriate precautions.

Fig. 4 demonstrates the appropriate lines for removal of the calvaria. The cut needs to be approximately as deep as the distance from the front of the skull to the lateral

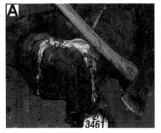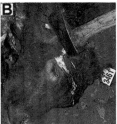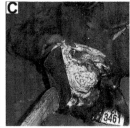

Fig. 4. The steps for opening the skull with an axe to expose the brain. (*A*) Cut across the face just dorsal to the lateral canthus then cut from the lateral canthus dorsal in front of the ear over to the poll, across the poll to the level of the opposite ear. (*B*) Using the blunt side of the single-bit axe, strike the edge of the cut bone between the lateral canthus and the ear at a 45° angle. (*C*) This will break the skull away from the brain.

canthus. Make sure the axe cuts are completely through the cranium. Using the blunt or hammer side of the single-bit axe, strike the cut edge of the cranium along the frontal crest at a 45° angle (see **Fig. 4**).

To remove the brain, cut the dura mater across the cerebral falx, the tough medial division of the dura. Extend this cut to allow the fingers to slide beneath the cerebrum. Using the necropsy knife, cut between the cerebrum and the cerebellum at the level of the pons and lift the cerebrum out of the cranium. Next, split the dura mater covering the cerebellum dorsally. Slide the tip of the necropsy knife behind the cerebellum into the spinal canal and cut across the spinal cord distal to the obex. Lift out the cerebellum and spinal cord, containing the obex.

Opening the Hide and Reflecting the Legs

Using a box cutter, cut along the underside of the jaw, over the larynx, and down the neck over the trachea. The incision should drift toward the animal's right foreleg axillary space. Continue the skin incision along the ventral thorax, crossing the costal cartilages and along the abdominal wall toward the right rear inguinal area. The incision across the thorax and abdomen will be lateral to the midline 3 to 6 inches (**Fig. 5**).

Do not cut the hide upward toward the scapula as the foreleg axillary space is passed. The hide is worth half of the value of the carcass to the renderer, and mutilating the hide reduces its value so much that many renderers will not pick up necropsied carcasses without charging a fee if the hide is damaged.

Reflect the rear leg before attempting to reflect the foreleg. To reflect the rear leg, cut the heavy muscles (adductor, semimembranosus, pectineus, and sartorius) that hold the coxofemoral joint in place. The round ligament will be easily identified and the joint examined (see **Fig. 5**).

The best approach to examining the stifle and hock joints is to start with the rear leg reflected and then skin along the inside of the leg from the stifle joint past the hock joint. To examine the stifle joint, cut along the side of the femoral trochlea and cut above the patella through its attachment to the quadriceps down to the femur. The patella will rotate over, yielding a great view to the stifle joint. To examine the hock joint, slide the necropsy knife between the extensor muscles and the tibia and cut the extensors loose below the stifle joint. Retracting the extensor muscles will allow the knife to be slide down to the hock joint, and then pull up the joint capsule, thus allowing one to cut open the joint capsule without invading the joint with the tip of the knife blade. This allows for cleaner joint sampling.

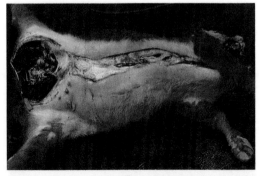

Fig. 5. Note the real leg is reflected while the foreleg remains unreflected. Working from the back side, continue to skin forward toward the foreleg. Lift the foreleg and cut through the latissimus dorsi holding the foreleg down.

Working from the back side, continue to skin the carcass toward the fore leg. When skinned to the level of the transverse processes and proximal rib attachments, the latissimus dorsi holding the foreleg down will be easily cut. Move to the sternal side of the animal and lift the foreleg, cutting the pectoral muscles. The foreleg should lay over with only minor fascia dissection.

Examining the Oral Cavity and Neck Structures

Incise along the side of the cheek, exposing the premolars and molars. This approach provides a good view of the oral cavity and allows for examination of molar eruption (**Fig. 6**). The first molar erupts in cattle at approximately 7 months of age and is in full wear at approximately 12 months.[4] This information can be useful when examining stocker and light feeder cattle.

To examine the tongue and larynx, slide the knife on the caudal side of the hyoid bones, feeling for the bend formed between the epihyoid and the ceratohyoid bones. The knife will generally cut the cartilage connection easily in younger animals. Shears can be used if needed.

Reflect the tongue while dissecting the larynx, trachea, and esophagus. Open the esophagus, larynx, and trachea down to the level of the thoracic inlet for examination. If a "bloat-line" observation is potentially important in the necropsy, this would be a good time to separate the esophagus from the trachea to the level of the thoracic inlet. Later in the necropsy, when the pluck is reflected over the first rib, the esophagus can be retracted through the thoracic inlet and its entire length can be examined.

Opening the Abdomen and Thorax

There are several acceptable ways to gain entry into the abdomen. The author generally starts by incising the abdominal wall along the greater curvature of the last rib, being careful not to incise the intestine. Once a hand-size hole is made, the author reverses the grip on the necropsy knife so the tip of the handle is forward, slides the hand into the abdomen with the knife handle leading the cutting edge, and incises the abdominal wall as the hand is advanced (**Fig. 7**). The incision is continued until the abdominal wall can be reflected.

The greater omentum is cut away, revealing the small intestine and allowing the abdominal viscera to shift away from the diaphragm, which is examined and cut free along its costal attachment. Using shears or an axe, cut across the distal ribs close to

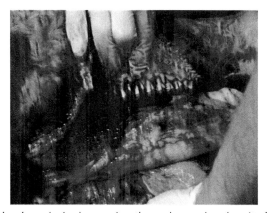

Fig. 6. The cheek has been incised, exposing the molars and oral cavity for examination.

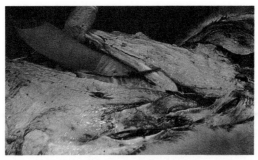

Fig. 7. Opening the abdomen by working with the hand inside and the knife blade pointing outside will help prevent puncturing loops of intestine.

the costochondral junctions. The ribs may be separated and manually reflected by breaking the costovertebral joint, or one can cut across the proximal ribs close to the costovertebral joints and reflect the entire plate of ribs forward off the top of the thoracic organs (**Figs. 8** and **9**). Leave the first rib intact. This will hold the thoracic organs in the carcass as it is winched onto the rendering truck. It is always a good idea to be considerate of both production personnel and those who work for the renderer.

Examining the Thoracic Cavity

First examine the pericardial sac and fluid. Detach the lung by cutting between the thoracic vertebra and aorta. Then dissect the dorsal lung free from the anterior thoracic to the diaphragm (**Fig. 10**). Next, free the caudal right lung lobe from the diaphragm by cutting the aorta, esophagus, and mediastinal reflections (right and left) between the pericardial sac and diaphragm. Continue detaching the pluck by cutting attachments between the pericardial sac and ventral thoracic. Reflect the lungs and heart forward over the first rib (**Fig. 11**).

Palpate the lung for abnormalities. Examine the tracheobronchial lymph nodes and airways. Examine the thoracic esophagus. The esophagus can be pulled through the thoracic inlet if a potential bloat line is of interest.

The heart's pericardium, myocardium, and endocardium are evaluated as the organ is opened. Start the examination with the right heart. Make an incision in the right ventricle just below the vena cava and extend the incision through the semilunar

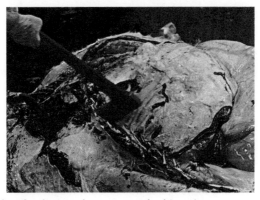

Fig. 8. Cut across the ribs close to the costovertebral junctions.

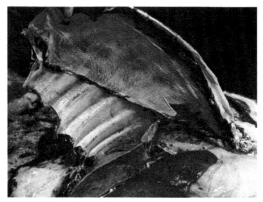

Fig. 9. After cutting across the ribs dorsally and the ventral costochondral junctions, reflect the rib plate forward.

valves. Extend the incision distally along the border of the right ventricular wall around its entire connection to the septal wall. This flaps the right ventricle and allows an excellent view of the tricuspid valve. To open the left ventricle, make an incision in the middle of the ventricle such that when opened, the 2 large papillary muscles will lay on either side of the incision. Cut across the ventricle just below the coronary grove. This forms a "T"-shaped incision, allowing the bicuspid valves to be examined. The left semilunar valves can be examined by extending the vertical incision into the aorta. These steps are illustrated from left to right in **Fig. 12**.

Examining the Abdominal Cavity

The small intestines can be fanned out or spread over the rumen for examination (**Fig. 13**). Autolysis generally makes opening the entire length of the intestine pointless.

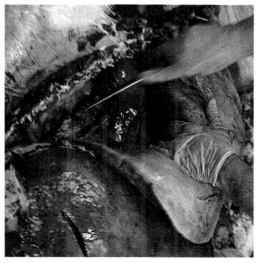

Fig. 10. To remove the lung and heart, start by dissecting the lung away from the thoracic vertebra. Continue dissecting the lung free from the diaphragm and the pericardial attachments from the sternum.

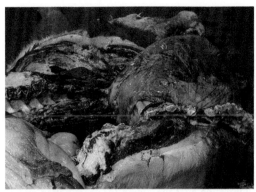

Fig. 11. Reflect the lung over the first rib. It allows for complete examination of the lung, associated lymph nodes, and heart.

However, mesenteric lymph nodes will retain their architecture longer than bowel and are useful in evaluating inflammatory changes. Always examine the ileocecal valve for signs of inflammation as could be associated with salmonellosis.

Although the small intestine is spread over the rumen, examine the right kidney and liver. Flip the small intestine over the transverse processes, exposing the small colon (**Fig. 14**), left kidney, bladder, distal colon, and rectum (if a female, their reproductive organs) for examination.

Make a palm-size hole in the rumen behind the anterior pillars. Reach in and find the ruminoreticular fold. Pull the fold to surface and examine the side next to the cranial sack for acidosis lesions or scars.

Palpate the abomasum, reticulum, and omasum for masses and normal texture. Reach under the anteroventral edge of the abomasum next to the diaphragm and grasp the spleen. Retract the spleen for examination. Open the abomasum to examine the surface for lesions such as ulcers, parasites, or scarring.

RECORDING OBSERVATIONS

The principal purpose of field necropsies is to gain information that may evaluate or influence production management decisions. Necropsy reports are intended to communicate the necropsy observations to others and to serve as a record that

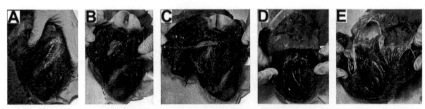

Fig. 12. The sequence represents the recommended steps for examining the heart. This approach allows for thorough examination of all valves and myocardial muscle structure. (*A*) The knife opens the right ventricle, allowing the incision (*B*) to extend into the outflow. (*C*) The right ventricle has been completely opened, allowing examination of the tricuspid valve. (*D*) Two incisions have been made in the left ventricle. One has been longitudinally and the other across the ventricle below the coronary grove. This exposes the bicuspid valve for examination. (*E*) The longitudinal incision has been extended through the aorta.

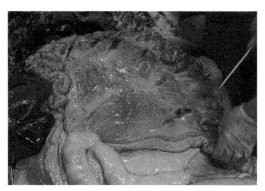

Fig. 13. Fan the small intestine over the rumen for examination and cut across the mesenteric lymph nodes.

can be used in production management. The brevity that many practice in our reports creates severe deficiencies in communication. There is a better way.

Necropsy Observations Check-Off Form

A form can be created that allows rapid highlighting of the circumstance and health management history, noting and checking off body systems involved, highlighting observations within each system examined, and summarizing tentative causes or diagnosis (**Fig. 15**). This is particularly beneficial when necropsies are performed by trained personnel instead of the veterinarian. A consistent set of digital photographs of each necropsy that includes the *animal's identification tag in each photograph* can be valuable when communicating with the off-site veterinarian, pathologist, or lawyer. The photograph taken may include the surface and opened view of the lung with the tracheobronchial lymph node, heart, kidney, and the small intestine with an associated mesenteric lymph node. A necropsy form for cattle can be divided into 3 parts: history, observations, and cause or diagnosis.

The history portion of the form should include the date, animal identification and description, environmental stress information, and health information. It may or may not include a vaccination history, but this could easily be added.

The observation portion of the form includes each body system and several observations that can be made in each body system. Users will likely be uncomfortable trying to limit their observations to the number available on a form. The quality and

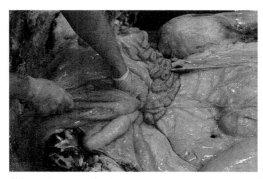

Fig. 14. Flip the small intestine over the transverse processes to expose the small colon and allow access to the distal colon, left kidney, bladder, and reproductive system.

Field Streaking a Blood Agar Plate
(needle aspirate inoculated with a bent 20 gage needle)

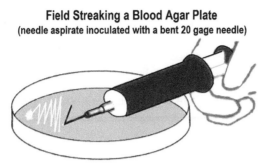

Fig. 15. Example of a "check-off" necropsy observation collection form.

quantity of information gathered will far exceed what is typically found in most practitioners brief necropsy reports.

The cause and diagnostic section of the form may include a series of boxes that allows one to numerically rank the observer's opinion of the importance of the body system involved and rank the suspected cause involved. The final portion of the form has a place for comments and suspected diagnosis.

The highlights of each necropsy can be kept in a simple Microsoft Excel spreadsheet or Microsoft Access (Redmond, WA, USA) database. This allows necropsy report forms to be easily searched for relationships between cases and production management decisions.

The form described in a Microsoft Word format can be downloaded from the University of Nebraska – Lincoln, Great Plains Veterinary Educational Center's Internet site (http://GPVEC.UNL.EDU) under "Griffin's Teaching Files."[5]

HANDLING, PACKAGING, AND SHIPPING DIAGNOSTIC SPECIMENS

Tissue specimen degradation is a serious issue that can severely handicap a diagnostic laboratory's ability to provide usable information. Histopathology specimens should be sliced thin, less than 7 mm, at the time they are collected. Intestine tissue samples are especially sensitive to crushing damage, and it is important to ensure the 10% formalin (3.7% formaldehyde) is in contact with the intestinal lining. If formalin is not available at the time of necropsy, keep the samples *cold and separated*. Most pathologists suggest taking samples from all major body systems with associated lymph nodes if changes are noted. More than 1 sample would be appropriate from the body system(s) that exhibited significant pathologic changes, including sections along the boundaries between normal and abnormal tissue.

Tissue samples collected for microbiology pose unique challenges. These specimens generally are not sliced as thin as are specimens for histopathologic examination and therefore are more prone to heat degradation. The bacteria in the specimen, targeted for both culture and contaminants, continue to grow. Contaminant bacteria may replicate faster and/or they may produce substances as they grow that inhibit the replication and subsequent recovery of the targeted bacterium. For this reason, the author frequently collects a needle aspirate of the tissue to culture and collects tissue specimens for laboratory microbiologist.

Needle aspirate collection for microbiology is a simple procedure that allows submission of an inoculated blood agar plate to the laboratory along with the other specimens. Starting cultures in the field improves the turnaround time and can improve the accuracy of diagnosis of some diseases. The author takes aspirates using a 10-mL syringe and a 20-gauge 1.5-inch needle. The author flames the needle using a butane lighter until it is red hot, then inserts it into the target tissue to be cultured. The hot needle should sear the surface and prevent contamination of the aspirate from surface contaminants. Aspirate fluid and tissue into the needle and syringe. After necropsy, the author sprays collected aspirates on blood agar plates. Next, bend the 1.5-inch needle in a 45° angle and flame the angle formed until sterile. Use the bent needle to streak the agar plate (**Fig. 16**). Tape the edges of the agar plates. Double bag each plate, and it is ready for shipping to diagnostic laboratory.

Date: _____ Yard, Pen/Lot & Animal ID: _____ Samples taken Yes / No

Sex (S-H-B/C) Breed (British-Zebu-Exotic-Dairy)   Weight: (<4, 4-6, 6-8, 8-10, >10)   Approx DOF: _____

Died Where (Receiving, Home, Hosp, Recovery)   Euthanized (Y / N)   Type stress (Heat-Shipping-Rain-Mud)

L temp: <40s, 50s, 60s, 70s   H temp: <60s, 70s, 80s, 90s, >100

Pull Dx _____   Previously Sick (N -Y: <30 or >30 days)

RxAB: Exc-Exl-Nax, Draxxin, Zactran, Micotil, Nuflor, Baytril, OTC, Pen, Amp, Sulfa, / Mass Med: (Y-N-U)

PHOTO Surface & Opened with ID in pic: Lung +LN, Heart, Liver, Kidney, Sm. Intestine +Mesenteric LN, Other

Place an "NE" next to body systems that NOT EXAMINED		
GENERAL CONDITION	**HEART**	**Reproductive**
BCS ( )	Outside infection	Infected
Fresh (F) or Rotten (R)	Inside infection	pregnant (early, mid, late)
	Bloody spots on surface	
SKIN	Enlarged	**JOINTS & BONES**
General hair loss or skin infection		Injury
Sinus injury or infection	**INTESTINE**	Infected
Mammary gland infected	Contents bloody	
	Lymph nodes large	**MUSCLES**
Oral Cavity Lesions (Y/N)	Infection	Neck – bloody
	Peritonitis	Back & side – blood spots
NECK	Obstructed	Hind leg – pale
Bad IV injection		Injection site
Dark blood filled neck	**LIVER**	Muscle injury
	Rotten big yellow spots	
ESOPHAGUS	General yellow color	**SPLEEN**
Ulcers or Erosions	Abscess	Swollen and full of blood
Edema (Parasites)	Migrating Flukes (black streaks)	
	Large Hard Congested (Nutmeg)	**Kidney (Lf /Rt)**
TRACHEA		Abnormal color (Pale / Dark)
Larynx lesion	**GALLBLADDER**	Rough with scars or streaks
Trachea Red or bloody	Enlarged	Bloody spots
Top thick & bloody	Bloody inside surface	Mushy rotten
Froth or fluid in lumen	Bile ducts-Flukes	Infection /Pus
		Bladder – red spots or infected
LUNG	**RUMEN RETICULUM-OMASUM:**	Urine – bloody or flocculent
Fluid around lung	Free Gas	
Lung collapsed	Froth	**BRAIN**
Lung fluid filled	Bloody spots on folds	Dark red and watery
Lung gas / emphysema	Ulcers	Slight pus on the bottom
Lung dark & hard	Traumatic adhesions	Small dark rotten areas
Lung abscesses		Injury
Lung stuck to ribs	**ABOMASUM:**	
Lung lymph node large & angry	Thick folds	**CANCER ... where?**
%Affected (<1/3,1/3-2/3,>2/3)	Ulcers	
Approx Age (<1, 1-3, >3 wks)	Thick with white spots	

CAUSE	U=Unknown	Rank Sys & Cause	Cause	Rank	Rank Sys & Cause	Cause	Rank	Rank Sys & Cause	Cause	Rank
C=Circulatory E=Enviom	F=Feed Relat	Gen Body			Skin / SubQ			Musculo-Skeletal		
I=Infectious M=Metabolic	Ne=Neoplasia	Respiratory			Circ / Hem / Lymp			Gastro-Intestinal		
P=Parasitic T=Trauma	Tx=Toxic	Urinary			Reproductive			Nervous		

General Comments &/or Diagnosis: _____

Fig. 16. Starting bacteriology culture shortly after the necropsy provides an additional opportunity for the diagnostic laboratory to make a better evaluation. In this illustration, a needle aspirate has been inoculated on a blood agar plate and the aspirating needle, after bending and heat sterilization, is used to streak the agar inoculum.

Important packaging and shipping definitions[6–8]

- Biologic substances, category B means any human or animal material being shipped for diagnostic purposes. *These specimens must have both a "Biologic Substance" label and a UN3373 diamond logo* (**Fig. 17**) *on the shipping container.* As noted, the "Infectious Substances" designation *does not apply* to diagnostic specimens that would be shipped to diagnostic laboratories. Appropriate labels are available online or from a state diagnostic laboratory.
- The 10% formalin used for animal diagnostic samples is a volume-per-volume mixture of 1 part 37% formaldehyde added to 9 parts water (with or without additional buffers). This dilution does not meet the US Department of Transportation's definition for a hazardous material under the Hazardous Materials Regulation; 49 CFR Parts 171–180[6] and is not regulated. Air transportation requirements additionally must meet the International Air Transport Association requirements. Currently, individual fixed specimen sample containers are kept to less than 30 mL or 1 ounce of 10% formalin; up to 33 of these individual containers, or less than 1 L total formalin, can be shipped by air transportation.[7]
- Regulatory agencies
  - US Department of Health and Human Services regulates the interstate shipment of etiologic agents.[6]
  - The US Department of Transportation regulates ground and air transportation of diagnostic specimens, infectious substances, medical waste, and chemical and radioactive materials (www.hazmat.com).[7]
  - Samples shipped by ground (courier, bus, postal service, etc.) follow the US Department of Transportation Code of Federal Regulations (49CFR)[7]
  - The International Air Transport Association, although not an agency, writes the requirements for all air transportation.[8]

Common carriers include Federal Express (fedex.com) and the US Postal Service (usps.com).

Shipping Good Management Practice[9–13]

- Use a sturdy reinforced container; Styrofoam (Dow Chemical, Midlan, MI, USA) boxes should be inside a cardboard box.
- Place coolant packs in Ziploc (S.C. Johnson & Son, Racine, WI, USA) bags in case of leakage or rupture.

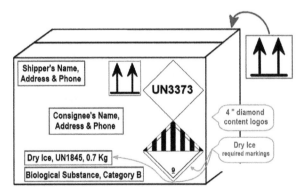

Fig. 17. This is an example of a properly labeled biologic substance "Category B" shipping container that contains dry ice. Note the weight of the dry ice is included on the label.

- Avoid overfilling liquid containers, don't exceed one-half of the container capacity.
- Whirl-Pak (Uline, Pleasant Prairie, WI, USA) bags are superior to Ziploc bags; twist-tie the metal strip after closing.
- Tape all rubber-stoppered tubes.
- Double check for potential leakage of all containers.
- Place all specimens inside a large plastic bag that contains sufficient absorbent (cat litter or paper towels) for all the fluid in the containers to be shipped should they be damaged during shipment.
- Avoid breakable specimen containers … if used, pad and double bag the container.
- Place paperwork in waterproof bag; Ziploc bags work best.
- If there are shipment questions, contact the carrier and/or laboratory.

Packaging Diagnostic Specimens (Biologic Substances, Category B)

Diagnostic specimens must be triple packed as follows:

- *Primary container* should be a screw cap tube, taped red top blood tube, or Whirl-Pak bag wrapped with the *tie ends twisted together. Ziploc bags are not suitable for liquid primary containers.*[9–12]
- *Secondary container* must be water-tight and have sufficient absorbent, such as paper towels, should the primary container leak or rupture.
- *Outer package* (*third layer of the specimen shipment container*) should be at least as durable as sturdy cardboard. Although Styrofoam is an excellent container; it should never be used as a shipping container without residing in a sturdy cardboard box. Styrofoam coolers are not acceptable as the exclusive outer container because of the potential for rupture if dropped or impacted in a transportation accident.
- USPS limits less than 1 L (1 L) liquid per primary container with total of less than 4 L or less than 4 kg solid per shipment. USPS requires a biohazard logo. Some carriers limit shipment to less than 0.5 L or less than 0.5 kg solids.
- Shipper's and consignee's contact information, including 24-hour telephone number, should be on the label (**Fig. 17**).
- Both a "Biologic Substance" label and a UN3373 diamond logo (see **Fig. 16**) should be on the outer shipping container.

BOTTOM LINE

Diagnostic specimens must be packaged in triple packaging consisting of[9–12]: (1) a primary container, such as a screw-cap tube or plastic bag; (2) a secondary container that must be watertight and contain sufficient absorbent to capture any leakage; (3) outer packaging that is of sturdy cardboard (do not use Styrofoam coolers as the outer container); and (4) a properly labeled shipping container (see **Fig. 17**).

Assume that specimens will travel in part by air, so meet International Air Transport Association shipping requirements (eg, *1 L of 10% formalin* per properly packaged sample container, or 30 mL per sample container if it includes formaldehyde of >10% concentration). Shipping with dry ice has a few additional requirements (see **Fig. 17**).[12] The outer shipping container must be marked with "Carbon Dioxide, Solid or Dry Ice" and the UN Identification Number "UN1845" and a Class 9 label.

REFERENCES

1. Federal Food, Drug, and Cosmetic Act (FD&C Act), Section 402(a)(1) or (2), CPG Sec. 675.400 Rendered Animal Feed Ingredients, Revised: 11/13/98. FDA, Washington, DC.

2. Jubb KV, Kennedy PC, Palmer N. 3rd edition. Pathology of domestic animals, vol. 3. San Diego (CA): Academic Press; 1985. p. 175–92.

3. Dyce KM, Sack WO, Wensing CJ. Textbook of veterinary anatomy. 3rd edition. Philadelphia: Saunders; 2002. p. 627–760.

4. Cropsey LM. Technical aspects of determining over-age in beef cattle. Proceedings of the American Association of Bovine Practitioners. Auburn, AL; 1974. p. 67–71.

5. Griffin DD. NecropsyDataBase_Classify&Photo2010Form_DGriffin.doc Griffin's Teaching Files. University of Nebraska – Lincoln, Great Plains Veterinary Educational Center's Internet site. Available at: http://gpvec.unl.edu/files/listsub.asp?path=/griffin/Necropsy.

6. Interstate shipment of etiologic agents. Code of Federal Regulations Title 42 Part 72, Interstate shipment of etiologic agents (Public Health). U.S. Government, Washington, DC: 65 FR 49908, August 16, 2000.

7. Hazardous materials regulations. Code of Federal Regulations Title 49 Subchapter C: hazardous materials regulations, Part 171, 172, 173, 175. Department of Transportation; Washington, DC: 76 FR 3345, Jan. 19, 2011. 73 FR 20772, April 16, 2008; FR 78634, Dec. 29, 2006.

8. Dangerous Goods Regulations. International Air Transport Association. IATA USA, 1201 F Street, N.W. Suite 650 Washington, DC 2012.

9. Safe operating procedures: shipping infectious substances. Lincoln (NE): University of Nebraska-Lincoln Department of Environmental Health and Safety; 2011.

10. Safe operating procedures: packaging and shipping hazardous materials / dangerous goods. Lincoln (NE): University of Nebraska-Lincoln Department of Environmental Health and Safety; 2010.

11. Safe operating procedures: shipping infectious substances with or without dry ice. Lincoln (NE): University of Nebraska-Lincoln Department of Environmental Health and Safety; 2011.

12. Safe operating procedures: shipping items with dry ice that are not otherwise dangerous goods. Lincoln (NE): University of Nebraska-Lincoln Department of Environmental Health and Safety; 2011.

13. Griffin DD, Shuck K. Packaging and shipping diagnostic samples. Clay Center (NE): University of Nebraska – Lincoln, Great Plains Veterinary Educational Center; 2011.

Ruminant Abortion Diagnostics

Larry D. Holler, DVM, PhD

KEYWORDS

- Ruminants • Abortion • Diagnostics

KEY POINTS

- Abortion rates vary between producers, production systems, and management styles, but in most situations, a rate much higher than 5% to 8% is usually deemed unacceptable.
- Costs of diagnostic services for abortion disease diagnosis can vary greatly among laboratories, but are often significant.
- Numerous improvements in test development have given the diagnostician powerful tools for etiologic diagnosis.
- Practitioners must understand the process and inherent limitations of abortion diagnostics, be able to help the producer determine if and when an investigation is warranted, and submit appropriate samples to a laboratory that specializes in diagnosis of reproductive failure in livestock.
- Successful abortion diagnosis in ruminants involves input from the producer, practitioner, and diagnostician.

Reproductive failure due to abortion disease remains a significant revenue drain in many ruminant livestock production systems. Abortion rates vary among producers, production systems, and management styles, but in most situations, a rate much higher than 5% to 8% is usually deemed unacceptable and worthy of investigation. Given currently high commodity prices for beef and lamb, the tolerated abortion rate may be much lower. Abortion storms such as were historically seen with infectious bovine rhinotracheitis (IBR), and more recently with *Neospora caninum*, can affect up to 10% to 40% of the pregnant animals and be devastating to the economic health of the producer.

Costs of diagnostic services for abortion disease diagnosis can vary greatly among laboratories, but are often significant. Implementing intervention strategies to impact ongoing abortion is usually limited, costly, and often of questionable efficacy.

The author has nothing to disclose.
Animal Disease Research and Diagnostic Laboratory, Veterinary and Biomedical Sciences Department, South Dakota State University, Box 2175, North Campus Drive, Brookings, SD 57007, USA
E-mail address: Larry.Holler@sdstate.edu

Vet Clin Food Anim 28 (2012) 407–418
http://dx.doi.org/10.1016/j.cvfa.2012.07.007   **vetfood.theclinics.com**

Preventive programs may need modifications, but in reality, most producers already have basic vaccination programs in place. The search for a definitive diagnosis, or even an "educated maybe," is often difficult in light of the many diagnostic challenges that are incumbent in abortion diagnostics. Therefore, practitioners must understand the process and inherent limitations of abortion diagnostics, be able to help the producer determine if and when an investigation is warranted, and submit appropriate samples to a laboratory that specializes in diagnosis of reproductive failure in livestock. Although ideal conditions rarely present themselves in the field, the practitioner and producer must be willing to work with the laboratory and diagnostician to find answers (if possible), hopefully in an economically feasible manner.

From a laboratory perspective, numerous improvements in test development have given the diagnostician powerful tools for diagnosis. Immunocytochemistry and new bacterial identification systems are rapid and highly sensitive. New multiplex polymerase chain reaction (PCR) formats are highly sensitive and allow rapid detection of multiple agents in a single test.[1] Histopathology, routine culture, fungal culture, fluorescent antibody (FA) tests, and virus isolation are still common and form the foundation of the approach to abortion diagnosis. Diagnostic laboratories are constantly evaluating new technologies for their ability to provide new diagnostic information. At the same time, diagnosticians must also be aware that these new techniques incur new costs that must eventually be passed on to the producer.

The development of new vaccines and improved vaccination strategies has reduced the impact of the once-major reproductive infectious diseases, such as IBR, bovine viral diarrhea virus (BVDV), brucellosis, and leptospirosis.[2,3] These once-major players are being replaced by an increase in opportunistic pathogens that seem to be emerging with changing production and management systems. The widespread use of total mixed rations and hay processing equipment in the upper Midwest ensures that any poor-quality feedstuff is incorporated into the total ration and consumed. The environmental bugs that used to be left in the moldy or rotten hay are now all but guaranteed entrance into the animal. The bottom line is that every year, significant financial losses from reproductive failure still occur despite vaccine and management improvements. The practitioner is faced with the dilemma of trying to find answers for these losses when often none exist. The diagnostician is often faced with trying to make a definitive diagnosis when none is possible. The cycle tends to repeat itself every year during "abortion season." Autolysis and incomplete submissions are known to be common challenges that face the diagnostician, but practitioners are limited by monetary constraints that dictate the diagnostic path to follow. Idiopathic abortion is a code phrase for "we just don't know," and is often the result of a variety of factors beyond the diagnostician's control. This article outlines some of the basic mechanisms and resulting pathology of abortion in ruminant livestock species and approaches for abortion diagnostic investigations that have evolved over the past 18 years of handling thousands of cases of reproductive wastage submitted to the diagnostic laboratory at South Dakota State University.

ABORTION VERSUS STILLBIRTH VERSUS LIVEBORN

The terminology of reproductive failure is often ignored by practitioners and producers. Embryonic mortality (up to 45 days) is often unnoticed and results in open animals or extended calving, lambing, and kidding intervals. These early fetal losses are associated with a wide range of physiologic, nutritional, environmental, and noninfectious causes that often go unrecognized.[4] Infectious causes of fetal loss during early gestation traditionally include *Tritrichomonas foetus, Leptospira borgpetersenii* serovar hardjo type hardjo-bovis (*Leptospira hardjo*), and BVDV.[5] In most circumstances, embryonic loss occurs without recovery of a conceptus. Abortion implies expulsion of a fetus before full term and viability outside of the uterus. Stillbirth or premature delivery is expulsion of a term fetus that is considered viable. Near-term fetuses, it is necessary to determine if the fetus was viable at expulsion or had been dead in utero. Antepartum death is characterized by variable degrees of autolysis, accumulations of blood-tinged fluids in body cavities, soft autolytic kidneys, and variable degrees of liquefaction of the brain. Tissues develop a uniform red-brown appearance from hemoglobin staining. Deaths associated with the parturition process are often less autolytic and display evidence of viability such as hemorrhage (functioning circulatory system), partial aeration of the lungs, meconium staining of the perineum and skin, swelling of the head and cervical region, subcutaneous edema, and fractures of ribs and limbs associated with the fetal expulsion process. Animals that have survived the birth process and died shortly after will have blood clots in umbilical vessels, aerated lungs, and minimal free fluid in body cavities.

Routes of Infection

The routes through which infectious agents reach the fetus include hematogenous spread through the placental–maternal interface where the placental chorioallantois attaches to the lining of the uterus at the caruncle. Additionally, ascending infection from the vagina through the cervical os can result in placental infection.[6] Infectious agents can colonize the placenta, penetrate into the amniotic fluid, and be swallowed by the fetus. Fungal organisms can penetrate the placenta and result in colonization of the fetal skin. Hematogenous spread results in passage through the liver and to the remaining tissue through the vascular system. Fetal pneumonia in these cases results in interstitial accumulation of organisms and inflammatory cells. For example, abortion associated with *Listeria monocytogenes* presents with massive bacterial growth, with organisms present in blood vessels in most fetal tissues. With this infectious species, inflammation is generally mild compared with the massive number of organisms present in tissues. Organisms can also enter the lung through the airways by inhalation of infected amniotic fluid. This amniotic fluid will often contain clumps of meconium, indicting advancing fetal stress caused by hypoxia.

Fetal hypoxia can result from maternal hypoxia, maternal circulatory system failure, or interference with oxygen transfer through the placental interface, most often associated with placentitis or premature placental separation. If possible, fetal compensatory mechanisms shunt blood to vital organs in an attempt to maintain normal oxygen levels. Fetal respiration increases in an attempt to compensate for hypoxia. This labored breathing is often associated with the aspiration of amniotic fluid. If the placenta is compromised because of slow-growing opportunistic bacteria or fungi, and the fetus is not immediately overwhelmed by the infection, the slowly advancing placental damage will suffocate the fetus from lack of oxygen or starve it from lack of nutrient transfer across the fetal maternal interface. If the fetus is not yet viable, abortion occurs; if the fetus is still viable but weakened from hypoxia, low nutrient transfer, and the possible deleterious effects of chronic infection, the outcome is often a stillborn or weak-born calf.

Clinical History

Appropriate collection and submission of samples for abortion diagnosis is critical for diagnostic success. A complete history, although often excluded on most submission forms, can be the first critical component to that success.

The following information that should be included:

- Size of the herd or flock, subgroups within the herd or flock, number of abortions (sporadic or epidemic), age of aborting animals, trimester in which abortions are occurring based on breeding dates or crown-rump measurements, recent purchases or whether it is a closed herd or flock, when and where any new additions were purchased from, previous reproductive history, natural service or artificial insemination, when the bulls or rams were pulled, exposure to other herds or flocks, and whether animals were clinically ill before or at the time of abortion
- Health management practices, including vaccination history, recent vaccinations, types of products, recent use of any modified live vaccines, recent treatments including feed-grade antibiotics, and treatments of clinical disease in the herd, flock, or affected individual animal
- Nutritional management, including types of feed; feed quality issues; feeding practices, including processing, feeding on the ground versus bunks, and trace mineral practices that may lead to deficiencies; potential toxic exposures to plants; nitrates/nitrites in feedstuffs; excessive minerals in feedstuffs (selenium); and water quality issues
- Environmental conditions, including heat or cold stress, overcrowding, and severe storm events

Unfortunately, nearly blank submission forms are often presented. Fortunately, the nervous producers or practitioners can often be consulted by telephone to fill in the gaps.

Sample Submission

Collection and submission of inappropriate or unsuitable samples is a disservice to the producer because it incurs needless costs and usually results in no useful information on which to base treatment or prevention strategies. Sample quality issues are a constant problem in abortion diagnostics. Aborted fetuses are often retained in utero, macerated, mummified, severely autolytic, partially eaten, covered in mud and manure, buried in bedding, frozen solid, or rotten from extreme heat. Superficial contamination can be rinsed away. Unfortunately, rotten is still rotten. Some samples are just unsuitable for evaluation. Gross lesions in abortion diagnostics are rare, and the submitted tissue is often soft, homogenous in color, and often bathed in red-black fetal fluid. Brain tissue is often liquefied and may pour out through the foramen magnum.

The whole fetus and complete placenta are considered ideal samples for submission if the laboratory is located in proximity to the producer. Fetuses are often at diagnostic laboratories at minimal or no additional charge. Crown-rump length is recorded as an estimation of fetal age, the overall stage of fetal development (**Table 1**) is noted, and the overall postmortem condition of the fetus is assessed.[7] External congenital anomalies are recorded and photographed (**Fig. 1**). Body or tissue weights are rarely collected unless a congenital disease is suspected and the fetus or individual organs are substantially smaller than expected. Necropsy procedures involve exposure of the thoracic and abdominal cavities, removal of the brain, and collection of appropriate tissues and body fluid, as listed in **Table 2**. These tissues can be collected easily in the field or veterinary clinic.

Placenta

The placenta is most significant tissue for abortion diagnosis. If unavailable, the probability of diagnosis is significantly reduced. A whole, intact placenta is rarely received

Table 1			
Estimation of fetal gestational age			
Crown-Rump Length (cm)	Age	Comparative Size	Physical Characteristics
1	30 d		
10	60 d	Mouse	
20	90 d	Rat	
30	120 d	Small cat	
45	150 d	Large cat	
60	180 d	Small dog	
80	210 d	Large dog	Hair around eyes, tail, muzzle
100	240 d		Hair on body, incisors slight eruption
>100	270 d		Near-term, incisors erupted

for examination. Often only a small portion of placenta is recovered and may be devoid of any cotyledonary structures. Rarely are these samples diagnostically useful. Histologic changes in placenta are often multifocal in distribution, requiring examination of multiple sections to give the diagnostician the best chance of detecting subtle areas of placental damage. Placentitis results in disruption of placental functions, including oxygen transport and exchange, nutritional support for the fetus, and hormone and growth factor production, which can affect normal parturition and fetal development. Chronic inflammation associated with release of cytokines and proinflammatory factors alters normal physiologic processes that occur at the fetal–maternal interface. Fetal macrophages within the placenta are rare in the early gestational fetus, but by 8 months' gestation, they have increased 10-fold. These macrophages are numerous within the allantoic stroma in areas of inflammation, and often seem to contain debris or organisms in their cytoplasm. Their role in cell defense against infectious agents and in dissemination of organisms is unknown.[8] The author believes that a significant number of stillborn or weak-born calves and lambs that are presented every late winter and spring are the result of placental dysfunction, often associated with chronic

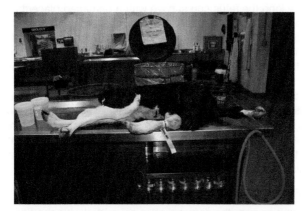

Fig. 1. Near-term bovine fetus with multiple congenital anomalies, including angular limb deformities and vertebral malformations. Suspected complex vertebral malformation in a Holstein calf.

Table 2
Samples to submit for ruminant abortion diagnosis

Whole fetus and placenta if proximity to laboratory is convenient; fresh (chilled) not frozen tissue samples, if entire fetus and placenta cannot be submitted:

Fresh[a]		Formalin-fixed[b]	
Lung (anterior lobes)	BV	Lung	HP
Kidney	VB	Kidney	HP
Liver	V	Liver	HP
Spleen	V	Spleen	HP
Heart	V	Heart	HP
Thyroid gland (ovine)	V	Thyroid (ovine)	HP
Placenta	BVM	Placenta	HP
		Skeletal muscle	HP
		Thymus	HP
		Brain	HP
		Ear notch	IHC

Fetal stomach content and bowel movement: collected with sterile syringe and submitted in snap cap tube
Fetal thoracic fluid/heart blood: collect with sterile syringe and submitted in snap cap tube
Ocular fluid for nitrate/nitrite analysis: collect with sterile syringe and submitted in snap cap tube
Maternal blood for serology[c]
Other: feed and water samples

Abbreviations: B, bacteriology; HP, histopathology; IHC, Immunohistochemistry; M, mycology; V, virology.

[a] Adequate fresh sample should be placed in leak-proof bags and chilled or frozen if delivery is delayed.

[b] Fix in adequate (10x) volume 10% buffered neutral formalin, submit in leak-proof sealed container.

[c] Maternal blood can be collected and serum harvested and saved frozen for future use.

placentitis. The outcome of pregnancy (abortion, stillborn, or weak-born) often depends on how long the fetus can survive with a damaged placenta.

A complete placenta is a large tissue, and placental lesions are often focal to multi-focal in distribution. Therefore, evaluation of a single small section of placenta may miss significant changes and result in a missed diagnosis. The author is constantly reminded by clients that the placenta often disappears shortly after birth for several reasons, but is satisfied if the client realizes that the diagnostic success rate is significantly reduced without the placenta. In the laboratory, the placenta is rinsed and cleared of contaminating debris and spread out for examination. It should be examined for gross changes, including the presence of exudate or thickening of intercotyledonary spaces or discoloration of cotyledons. The normal placenta is thin and transparent in the intercotyledonary areas, and the cotyledons are dark red-brown. The size and distribution of cotyledons should be noted.

Maternal and Fetal Serology

Single serum samples from the dam are often submitted with abortion investigations, but they are usually of little value in abortion diagnosis. Positive serology for an individual animal at best indicates exposure to a specific agent or antigens to a specific agent in the form of vaccine. Separating the 2 responses is often impossible. Knowledge of vaccination history, types and brands of vaccine used, and baseline serologic data from the specific laboratory performing the test is crucial to any serologic interpretation. In many laboratories, a positive serology result only means the animal has mounted a detectable immune response to the agent, and cannot separate actual exposure from vaccination. Most of the opportunistic infections, including environmental bacteria and fungi, do not have validated serologic tests. Many infectious agents stimulate titer increases that predate expulsion of the fetus. Therefore, using paired serum samples on individual animals to detect changes in titers is also rarely useful for demonstrating evidence of specific abortion agents. A serologic profile comparing aborted animals with normal controls is more often recommended. Serologic profiling on a significant number of animals in a herd may provide data on vaccination status for a given antigen and suspected exposure based on markedly elevated titers in the aborts versus the normal controls. Fetal serology may be useful in some instances. If the fetus is old enough to be immunocompetent, fetal immunoglobulin G (IgG) levels can be significantly elevated in fetal fluids in some infectious abortions. If IgG is elevated, then individual serologic tests can be performed as appropriate.[9] For example, indirect FA is a useful serologic test to detect antibody to *Toxoplasma gondii*. In *N caninum* abortions, fetal and neonatal serology was used to detect in utero infections in aborted fetuses or precolostral calves.

Diagnostic approach
When conducting abortion diagnostic workups, most laboratories tend to perform a standard battery of tests to cover the major bacterial, viral, fungal, and protozoal abortion diseases for the species submitted. Numerous excellent reviews on the complete list of potential agents are available and recommended for review.[9–11] History and gross examination may indicate a particular agent, but in practice, following a standard abortion protocol and performing additional tests as the investigation warrants is more practical. Ideally, one could test for every possible agent on each case, but financial considerations dictate that the diagnostic tests should be ordered selectively.

Bacterial infections
Most bacterial causes of abortion are opportunistic pathogens. These organisms are not infectious, and are common inhabitants of the host or its environment. These bacteria gain entrance to the bloodstream of the dam and occasionally introduce an infection in the placenta. *Arcanobacterium pyogenes* and *Bacillus* spp, followed by *Escherichia coli*, *Histophilus somni*, *Pasteurella* spp, *Listeria* spp, *Staphylococcus* spp, *Streptococcus* spp, and basically any other bacteria that can find its way into the bloodstream, can be opportunistic pathogens. These opportunists are usually associated with sporadic abortions, unless specific risk factors give a particular organism the chance to affect multiple animals. Cattle with abscesses or a history of feet problems seem to be affected by *A pyogenes*. Cattle exposed to processed bales with a great deal of soil-associated spoilage can have increased problems with *Bacillus* spp. *Listeria* spp is usually associated with poorly fermented silage feeding.

Most opportunists can cause abortion at any stage of gestation, but most are associated with late second to third trimester abortions. Gross lesions are rare but can include exudate on the placenta surface, or possibly increased fluid in body cavities, occasionally with fibrin. Histologic lesions include suppurative fetal pneumonia, mild perivascular inflammation in the epicardium and, to a lesser-extent myocardium, increased portal inflammatory cells in liver, and inflammatory cell pooling in blood vessels in the brain and other tissues. A variable severe, multifocal, necrotizing, and suppurative placentitis is a common lesion if adequate placenta is examined. Numerous intralesional bacteria are often observed histologically, especially in the case of *A pyogenes*–induced abortion. Bacterial culture of these organisms is usually straightforward, until one realizes that rarely do autolyzed fetuses yield pure growth of a single organism.

Campylobacter jejuni, *C fetus* subspecies *fetus*, and *Salmonella* spp are similar to *A pyogenes* in that numerous intracellular bacterial colonies are usually evident in sections of placenta, often associated with vigorous inflammation. These organisms are normal or transient inhabitants of the dam's intestinal tract and travel to the placenta during periods of bacteremia. *Campylobacter* spp and *Salmonella* spp are more commonly associated with abortions in sheep. Gross lesions, if present, are confined to the placenta and include accumulation of exudate or discoloration of cotyledons. Special culture media is required for *Campylobacter* spp, but *Salmonella* spp grows rapidly on conventional media. Brucellosis associated with *Brucella abortus* and other *Brucella* spp is rare in the United States. The most common member of this genus, *B ovis*, the agent associated with ram epididymitis, has been rarely associated with abortion in sheep. Serologic monitoring tests are available to detect cattle that have been exposed to *B abortus*. Special culture media is usually recommended for *Brucella* spp; however, culture specifically for this organism is not routinely attempted unless brucellosis is suspected.

Multiple species, serovars, and types of leptospira, including hardjo type hardjo-bovis, *pomona*, *icterohaemorrhagiae*, *grippotyphosa*, and most likely many others, can be involved in bovine embryonic loss and abortion.[12] Specific gross and histologic lesions have been described historically, but leptospira-induced abortions are so infrequent today that many diagnosticians would not recognize them. In the upper Midwest, the near-universal use of multivalent vaccines for *Leptospira* spp have significantly reduced its diagnosis associated with abortions in cattle. Culture of this organism is not practical because of time and cost constraints. Microscopic detection through dark-field examination of fetal fluids or silver-stained histologic sections is occasionally used, although the sensitivity of the techniques is low. A common technique, FA staining of kidney homogenates with multivalent antisera, is frequently used. Again, the sensitivity may be low, especially with host-adapted *Leptospira* spp, such as harjo type harjo-bovis. New PCR tests are currently in use and have the benefit of speed, specificity, and sensitivity. The PCR format is routinely used to detect carrier cows that shed the harjo-bovis organism in urine, and is becoming more common for detecting leptospira organisms in abortions.

Chlamydophila abortus associated with enzootic abortion in ewes is a significant cause of abortion in range sheep flocks, or farm flocks that buy range ewes for replacements. Gross lesions include thickening of the intercotyledonary spaces around affected cotyledons. Histologic lesions are most common in the placenta and, to a lesser degree, the liver. Placental lesions include a suppurative and necrotizing placentitis with marked stromal thickening and inflammation. The liver will rarely contain multifocal areas of necrosis. Diagnosis is accomplished routinely through immunocytochemistry of affected placenta. Serologic methods can detect specific antibody to *C abortus* in fetal thoracic fluid or heart blood. Although this organism can be cultured in embryonated eggs or in cell culture, very few laboratories still attempt isolation. PCR is available for *C abortus* at some laboratories, although the advantage PCR over immunohistochemistry is questionable in most routine circumstances.

The role of *Ureaplasma* spp and the agent associated with epizootic bovine abortion in bovine abortion seems to be significant in some geographic regions. Most laboratories do not routinely screen for these agents unless requested or lesions are present.

Viral Infections

Viral causes of abortion include bovine herpesvirus type 1, the cause of IBR, BVDV, and, to a lesser extent, bovine herpesvirus type 4 (BHV-4). Numerous references are available that describe these agents in detail.[2,5,9–11] IBR-associated abortions have decreased dramatically since the introduction of effective vaccination procedures. Recently, increased numbers of IBR abortions have been reported in unvaccinated or questionably vaccinated cows exposed to modified live vaccines during gestation. Gross and histologic lesions are commonly observed with IBR and can include pale foci in the liver that correspond with the multifocal necrotizing lesions that are present in several fetal tissues, including liver, lung, and spleen. Similarly, the incidence of BVDV has also decreased in the past several years, most likely because of increased vaccination. BHV-4 is considered an opportunistic viral pathogen and its role in abortion is difficult to determine. Diagnostic procedures for viral abortion agents vary among laboratories. Fluorescent antibody tests are rapid and usually of acceptable sensitivity. Virus isolation is considered a tried and true method, especially for discovery of new agents, but it is very expensive and time-consuming, and requires technical expertise. The advantage of virus isolation is that an isolate is available for further study or vaccine production at the end of the procedure. Molecular PCR-based tests have replaced other techniques in many laboratories because of their speed, specificity, and sensitivity. Multiplex PCR is currently available for IBR and BVD. Other viruses have been reported in certain geographic regions as causes of abortion and congenital anomalies. This group includes many arthropod-borne viral agents, such as bluetongue and Cache Valley virus.[13] Other viruses in the group are not routinely found in the United States, or require special diagnostic procedures performed at reference laboratories. Congenital anomalies can be associated with early bluetongue virus, Cache Valley virus, or BVDV infections.

Mycotic Infections

Mycotic abortion is common worldwide. The common agents include *Aspergillus fumigatus*, *Aspergillus* spp, *Candida* spp, and a variety of environmental species.[14,15] These organisms are ubiquitous saprophytes in the environment and often increase in numbers in moldy feedstuffs or bedding. Abortions usually occur when cattle are fed high concentrations of moldy stored or processed feedstuffs. The conidia from these organisms enter the respiratory tract or digestive tract, gain entrance into the bloodstream, and spread to the uterus and placenta. Gross lesions include thickening and roughening of cotyledons and intercotyledonary spaces. Lesions are often localized and may not be present if only a small portion of placenta is submitted. Histologic lesions, if present, will confirm a severe necrosuppurative placentitis and stromal arterial vasculitis. Fungal hyphae are often associated with these necrotic lesions.

Mycotic abortion can be diagnosed using fluorescent potassium hydroxide (KOH) staining procedures on placental scrapings to allow visualization of fungal elements. Special histochemical stains are also useful for histologic identification of fungal elements. Culture of fungal organisms from stomach content and placenta requires special media with added antibiotics to suppress bacterial growth. When a mixed growth of fungal organisms is isolated, the significance of the results should be questioned, but not dismissed. Multiple fungal species are often present in feed stuffs, and therefore dual infections cannot be completely eliminated as a possible diagnosis. If any particular fungal organism is isolated in heavy growth, or isolated in heavy growth from fetal stomach content and placenta and compatible placental lesions exist, then causality can be considered.

Protozoa

Protozoal agents associated with abortion include *N caninum*, *T gondii*, and *T feotus*.[16] *N caninum* is vertically transmitted from dam to congenitally infected normal offspring, and horizontally transmitted through ingestion of infective oocysts shed by the canine definitive host. Epidemic abortions were more common historically when most cattle were naïve to infection. The most common presentations associated with *N caninum* today are sporadic or endemic abortions. The dam is clinically normal, and most abortions occur between 5 and 7 months' gestation. Compatible lesions include multifocal necrosis and gliosis, and nonsuppurative epicarditis, myocarditis, and myositis. Occasionally, similar focal lesions are present in other tissues. Immunohistochemistry is used for detecting the organism in the context of the histologic lesion. PCR and several serologic tests are also available for diagnosis. Caution should be used if lesions are very mild or nontypical, because most calves born to seropositive dams will be congenitally infected, and the abortion could have been caused by other agents.

T gondii is similar to neosporosis but is primarily a problem in sheep and goats. The definitive host is the cat, and infective oocysts are usually consumed in contaminated feed stuffs. Mummification is common in *Toxoplasma*-induced abortion, and fetuses of various stages of development are often presented (**Fig. 2**). Histologic lesions include multifocal necrosis and gliosis in the brain and a nonsuppurative epicarditis. Oocysts of *T gondii* can occasionally be observed in routine histologic sections. Immunohistochemistry can improve detection of the organisms if needed. Indirect FA procedures can accurately detect antibodies specific for *Toxoplasma* in fetal fluids from aborted lambs or kids.

T foetus is most often associated with early embryonic death and early abortions in cattle. The organism can be cultured in special media from carrier bulls and occasionally from infected cows or recovered fetuses. PCR techniques have also been developed. In aborted fetuses, a mixed pneumonia is present, and occasionally protozoa compatible with *T foetus* can be found. Immunohistochemistry is available for diagnosis in fixed tissue.

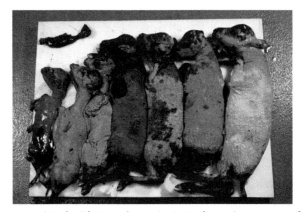

Fig. 2. Abortions associated with toxoplasmosis. Note the various stages of fetal development. All fetuses came from a single Finnsheep ewe that died from complications related to pregnancy toxemia.

Noninfectious Abortion

Noninfectious causes of abortion are often lumped together and include a variety of genetic, nutritional, and environmental factors associated with reproductive failure. This category is often a catch-all and is often overlooked in most diagnostic scenarios. Genetic causes of early embryonic mortality often go unnoticed. Embryonic loss associated with chromosomal defects or lethal mutations are rarely detected. Obvious congenital anomalies that present at birth often fit in 1 of 2 categories. The first includes animals with established genetic conditions, often with known genetic defects and testing strategies to eliminate the trait from the breed. The second and most common includes all other animals with a congenital anomaly. Caution is warranted in using the word *genetic* too early when investigating congenital malformations.[17] Many of the animals involved in these situations are extremely valuable, and data must be collected carefully and thoroughly before reaching any conclusion. Most nongenetic causes are probably still unknown, but nutritional factors, toxic plants, chemical exposure, and viruses should be considered as possible suspects. Toxic plant exposure during the first trimester can result in limb deformity, cleft palate, and spinal column abnormalities. Alkaloid-producing plants, such as the lupines, have been proven experimentally to cause malformations. Similar evidence exists for poison hemlock.[18] Exposure to mycotoxins has been suggested to contribute to limb and jaw anomalies. The challenge is determining which potentially toxic plant was present during the summer when the fetus was at 60- to 80-days' gestation when one is examining a calf submitted to the laboratory in March when 2 feet of snow are covering the ground. Nutritional factors, including trace mineral, vitamins, protein, and energy, can contribute to increased fetal loss and poor postnatal survival. Although many of these causal links are difficult to prove, the possibility of a nutritional component should be considered, if for no other reason than to give the producer the opportunity to evaluate and correct nutritional problems before they get worse. Exposure to parasiticides or other chemicals have been reported to have deleterious effects on fetal development, although the data are incomplete.

If genetic problems are suspected, diagnosticians should ensure they are dealing with purebred animals, offspring from a single sire, or offspring from very closely related sires, and that the defect occurs in expected frequencies. In reality, most genetic conditions that result in lethal outcomes in popular breeds cannot be hidden forever.

SUMMARY

Successful abortion diagnosis in ruminants involves input from the producer, practitioner, and diagnostician. Unfortunately, despite best efforts, many investigations still result in a diagnosis of idiopathic abortion. If this diagnosis is made after a complete and systematic investigation of appropriate and reasonably preserved samples, some comfort can be taken that practitioners and diagnosticians did their best for the benefit of the producer. As new diagnostic technology is developed for abortion diseases, hopefully the best will only get better.

DEDICATION

This work is dedicated to the late Dr Clyde Kirkbride, Professor, South Dakota State University, Animal Disease Research and Diagnostic Laboratory. Clyde was my mentor and friend. His desk and file cabinet, which is filled with a career's worth of knowledge on abortion disease in all species, still sit in my office. I keep them there as a reminder of his legacy and contribution to the field of abortion diagnosis. He was truly a pioneer.

REFERENCES

1. Tramuta C, Lacerenza D, Zoppi S, et al. Development of a set of multiplex standard polymerase chain reaction assays for the identification of infectious agents from aborted bovine clinical samples. J Vet Diagn Invest 2011;23:657–64.
2. Kirkbride CA. Viral agents and associated lesions detected in a 10-year study of bovine abortions and stillbirths. J Vet Diagn Invest 1992;4:374–9.
3. Kirkbride CA. Bacterial agents detected in a 10-study of bovine abortions and stillbirths. J Vet Diagn Invest 1993;5:64–8.
4. Kastelic JP. Noninfectious embryonic loss in cattle. Vet Med 1994;6:584–9.
5. Bon Durant RH. Selected diseases and condition associated with bovine conceptus loss in the first trimester. Theriogenology 2007;68:461–73.
6. Miller RB. A summary of some of the pathogenetic mechanisms involved in bovine abortion. Can Vet J 1977;18:87–9.
7. Mickelsen WD, Evermann JF. In utero infections responsible for abortion, stillbirth, and birth of weak calves in beef cows. Vet Clin North Am Food Anim Pract 1994; 10(1):1–14.
8. Schlafer DH, Fisher PJ, Davies CJ. The bovine placenta before and after birth: placental development and function in health and disease. Anim Reprod Sci 2000;60–61:145–60.
9. Anderson ML. Infectious causes of bovine abortion during mid-to late gestation. Theriogenology 2007;68:474–86.
10. Barr BC, Anderson ML. Infectious diseases causing bovine abortion and fetal loss. Vet Clin North Am Food Anim Pract 1993;9(2):343–68.
11. Givens MD, Marley MS. Infectious causes of embryonic and fetal mortality. Theriogenology 2008;70:270–85.
12. Ellis WA. Leptospirosis as a cause of reproductive failure. Vet Clin North Am Food Anim Pract 1994;10(3):463–78.
13. Ali H, Ali AA, Atta MS, et al. Common, emerging, vector-borne and infrequent abortogenic virus infections of cattle. Transbound Emerg Dis 2012;59:11–25.
14. Knudtson WU, Kirkbride CA. Fungi associated with bovine abortion in the northern plains states (USA). J Vet Diagn Invest 1992;4:181–5.
15. McCausland JP, Slee KJ, Hirst FS. Mycotic abortion in cattle. Aust Vet J 1987;6: 129–32.
16. Anderson ML, Barr BC, Conrad PA. Protozoal causes of reproductive failure in domestic ruminants. Vet Clin North Am Food Anim Pract 1994;10:439–61.
17. Steffen D. Investigating congenital diseases of calves. Proceeding handout for the James Bailey Herd Health Conference. Brooking (SD); 2010. p. 56–68.
18. James LF, Panter KE, Stegelmeier BL, et al. Effects of natural toxins on reproduction. Vet Clin North Am Food Anim Pract 1994;10(3):587–603.

Laboratory and Postmortem Diagnosis of Bovine Respiratory Disease

Jeff L. Caswell, DVM, DVSc, PhD[a],*, Joanne Hewson, DVM, PhD[b],
Đurđa Slavić, DVM, MSc, PhD[c], Josepha DeLay, DVM, DVSc[c], Ken Bateman, DVM, MSc[d]

KEYWORDS

- Postmortem examination • Laboratory diagnostic investigation
- Bovine respiratory disease complex • Enzootic pneumonia • Bovine respiratory syncytial virus
- *Dictyocaulus viviparus* • Acute phase proteins

KEY POINTS

- A routine diagnostic investigation of bovine respiratory disease should be comprehensive and robust, allowing identification of common but also unexpected diseases. This may require examination of multiple animals, sampling for histopathology and microbiologic testing, and storing samples pending the outcome of initial tests.

- An effective and concise clinical history is an essential element of any laboratory submission. In addition to the clinical diagnosis, it must include specific clinical observations that help the diagnostician to interpret the laboratory findings.

- Postmortem examination reveals the distribution and texture of lesions, indicating one or more morphologic patterns of lung disease, and thereby suggesting causes of disease and providing tissues for confirmatory testing. To be relevant, the animals examined must be representative of the clinical problem, early in the course of disease, and untreated if possible; the multiple tissues analyzed should focus on primary lesions but represent the spectrum of changes observed. Important diagnoses will be overlooked if the examination does not include the upper respiratory tract, caudal bronchi, pulmonary arteries, and heart, and nonspecific changes in the lungs must be recognized.

- Serology, although limited by the time needed for convalescent sampling, is an effective and sensitive method of establishing the cause of respiratory disease outbreaks.

- The investigation is doomed if the animals sampled are not representative of the disease problem, if they are sampled too late in the disease course, if too few or inappropriate tissues are sampled, if specimens become autolyzed or undergo freeze-thaw damage, or if vaccination or maternal antibody interferes with detection of the pathogen.

- Laboratory testing, such as measurement of serum haptoglobin, is useful as an indicator of inflammatory disease and a measure of disease severity.

The authors are supported by the Natural Sciences and Engineering Research Council of Canada (NSERC), the Ontario Cattleman's Association, the Agricultural Adaptation Council, and the Ontario Ministry of Agriculture, Food, and Rural Affairs.
The authors have nothing to disclose.
[a] Department of Pathobiology, Ontario Veterinary College, University of Guelph, Guelph, Ontario N1G 2W1, Canada; [b] Department of Clinical Studies, Ontario Veterinary College, University of Guelph, Guelph, Ontario N1G 2W1, Canada; [c] Animal Health Laboratory, University of Guelph, Ontario N1G 2W1, Canada; [d] Department of Population Medicine, Ontario Veterinary College, University of Guelph, Guelph, Ontario N1G 2W1, Canada
* Corresponding author.
E-mail address: jcaswell@uoguelph.ca

Respiratory disease continues to be a major cause of clinical disease, mortality, production loss, and reduced carcass quality. Because the various causes of bovine respiratory disease (BRD) have overlapping clinical manifestations, pathologic and laboratory investigations are often required in those cases for which a specific diagnosis is required. A specific diagnosis is useful to direct antimicrobial or anthelmintic therapy, vaccination programs, and biosecurity practices and to satisfy the curiosity and concern of producers and veterinarians.

This review uses 4 cases to illustrate diagnostic approaches to the laboratory diagnosis of BRD, recognizing that the clinical, pathologic, and microbiologic aspects of the investigation each contribute key pieces of information. Some aspects are described in detail elsewhere, including descriptions of specific diseases,[1–6] neonatal respiratory distress syndrome,[7,8] necropsy technique, interpretation of necropsy findings,[9,10] sample submission to laboratories,[11,12] and interpretation of antimicrobial susceptibility testing.[13,14]

CASE 1: AN OUTBREAK OF RESPIRATORY DISEASE IN DAIRY CALVES

An outbreak of respiratory disease occurred in an unvaccinated 350-cow dairy herd in December. Temperatures had been unseasonably warm, above freezing, then fell to −10°C overnight. Signs of disease appeared suddenly the following day. Adult cows were not affected. The outbreak involved 4- to 7-month-old calves kept as replacement stock. There was no history of recent introductions to the herd. At the time of examination, 30 calves of the group of 60 were affected, and 2 died as a result of respiratory distress. A necropsy examination performed by the practitioner revealed subcutaneous and pulmonary emphysema. The entire lung was firmer than normal. The cranioventral 70% of the lungs were darker red than the also-firm dorsocaudal lung.

Before embarking on an expensive diagnostic investigation, there is merit in reflecting on the objectives and the questions that might reasonably be answered. The goals vary considerably depending on the production system and the particular circumstances of each case. For respiratory disease involving beef cattle that have recently arrived to a feedlot, the important questions may be:

- Does the problem involve one or several diseases?
- Does the problem represent the usual occurrence of shipping fever pneumonia or something more unusual and unexpected?
- Are the health protocols for processing calves at arrival and adaptation to the feedlot working adequately?
- Is the age of the lesions consistent with the apparent timing of the clinical disease?

In contrast, the goal in this unexpected outbreak of disease in a group of dairy calves is to establish the exact cause to efficiently control the outbreak and institute changes to prevent future occurrences.

The major causes of respiratory diseases of cattle in North America, along with a summary of gross lesions and method of diagnosis, are listed in **Table 1**. Neonatal respiratory distress syndrome is a clinically distinct entity with multiple causes and is described elsewhere.[7,8] In this case, an outbreak of viral respiratory disease was considered most likely, but bacterial pneumonia or lungworm should also be considered.

The merits of the various diagnostic options are outlined in **Table 2**. The diagnosis in this case was based on necropsy examination of the calf that died, with laboratory testing of samples obtained at necropsy. Serologic investigation would have been a reliable method to reach the same diagnosis, albeit with the limitations that the results would not be known for several weeks, and laboratory costs could be higher. A third option would involve laboratory testing of samples obtained from live animals, such as nasal swabs or transtracheal washes. Although this can achieve a rapid diagnosis and has the flexibility of being based on few or many samples, it is a riskier option because most respiratory viral infections are transient, and testing therefore requires collection of samples early in the course of disease. Practitioners may not examine the herd until this early stage of infection has passed, whereas in large or extensively managed groups it may not be known which animals have most recently developed disease.

Key elements of the postmortem examination are outlined in **Box 1**. Veterinarians are faced with too many respiratory diseases to remember the features of each, so classification of lung diseases into morphologic patterns is helpful for diagnostic recognition of diseases, for understanding the pathogenesis and relationships between cause and clinical signs, and for predicting the chronic sequelae that may be seen in survivors. Pathologists vary in their exact categorization of pulmonary lesions and in the terminology applied, but the following system is broadly used. The main morphologic patterns, gross appearances, and causes are summarized in **Table 3** and illustrated in **Fig. 1A–H**).

Postmortem examination of the 2 calves that died revealed subcutaneous and pulmonary interlobular emphysema, increased weight of the lungs, and rubbery firmness of the cranioventral 70% of the lung (see **Fig. 1D** for similar lesions, from a different case). The emphysema, although dramatic, is a nonspecific consequence of respiratory distress, but the modestly increased texture of the cranioventral lung along with the clinical findings supports the possibility of viral bronchointerstitial pneumonia. Laboratory confirmation of the diagnosis was desirable in this case, based on the magnitude of the outbreak and the potential impact on future disease prevention strategies in the herd.

A concise but helpful clinical history is the foundation of the laboratory investigation. In the context of BRD, key features of the clinical history are summarized in **Table 4**. The clinical features just described were critical in guiding the diagnostic investigation that followed. Conversely, it is depressingly apparent in other cases that a poor or missing history results in inappropriate testing, errors in interpretation, and failure to effectively relate the pathologic findings to the clinical picture.

Boxes 2 and **3** outline considerations for tissue sampling from necropsy cases. Ideally, tissues should be collected from multiple animals that are reliably representative of the disease problem in the herd, early in the disease course, and not treated. This is often impossible for small herds of valuable animals, for which necropsy-based investigations must rely on the few animals that have died despite attempted therapy. In such cases, histopathologic examination often reveals lesions that suggest viral or bacterial pneumonia, yet the specific pathogen cannot be identified because it has been eliminated by the immune response or antimicrobial therapy. The lung is vast, and multiple (3–5) samples harvested from the various areas will increase the frequency of diagnosis. Foci of caseous necrosis are ideal for detection of *Mycoplasma bovis*, and granulomas are sites of *M bovis* infection, but abscesses are of no value in identifying the primary bacterial pathogen.

Histologically, in the present case, bronchiolar epithelium was thinned and irregular (bronchiolar necrosis); neutrophils, fibrin, and proteinaceous edema fluid packed the alveoli (bronchopneumonia), type II pneumocytes lined alveoli in a few areas (alveolar damage), and interlobular septa were emphysematous. These findings were interpreted as bronchointerstitial pneumonia suggestive of viral pneumonia and as

Table 1
Causes of BRD

Cause	Gross Lesions	Laboratory Diagnosis
Pasteurellaceae: *M haemolytica*, *Histophilus somni*, and *Pasteurella multocida*; *Mannheimia varigena*, and *Bibersteinia trehalosi*	Cranioventral reddening and firm to hard consolidation; may have irregularly shaped nonfriable foci of coagulation necrosis, interlobular edema (marbling), or fibrinous pleuritis	Histopathologic examination, bacterial culture of consolidated lung near the border with unaffected lung Live animal: clinical findings, response to treatment, ± culture of transtracheal wash
M bovis	Cranioventral reddening and collapse or consolidation, with round dry friable foci of caseous necrosis (see **Fig. 1A, B**).	Histopathology, IHC [a]Culture or RT-PCR[b] identifies *M bovis* but does not clarify the role in disease
Histophilus somni pleuritis	Fibrinous pleuritis, with or without consolidation of lung tissue (see **Fig. 1G**)	Culture of pleural exudate ± kidney, spleen, joints
Secondary or opportunistic bacterial pathogens: *Arcanobacterium pyogenes*, *Streptococcus* spp, etc	Cranioventral bronchopneumonia, abscesses, and/or bronchiectasis	Bacterial culture, but identifying the pathogen is not clinically useful
IBR (BHV-1)	Nasal cavity and trachea: multifocal to confluent erosions, covered with fibrin or necrotic debris Distinguish from expectorated lung exudate	Acute stage: VI,[b] PCR, or IHC Live animal: serologic investigation (acute and convalescent); or VI or PCR from nasal swabs
Viral pneumonia: BRSV, BCV, BHV-1, BPI3V	Cranioventral lung is red-purple and slightly firm-rubbery; dorsocaudal lung is similar with edema ± emphysema (see **Fig. 1D**) Cranial lung may have bronchopneumonia if there is secondary bacterial infection	Acute stage: PCR, IHC, VI, or antigen-capture ELISA (BRSV is labile and difficult to isolate), and RT-PCR is more sensitive[15] BCV isolation requires special HRT-18 cell lines[1] Live animal: serology (acute and convalescent); or VI or PCR using nasal swabs
Infection with BVDV or the viruses listed as predisposing causes of bacterial pneumonia	Cranioventral lung is red and firm-to-hard as a result of bacterial bronchopneumonia; dorsocaudal lung is normal or slightly firm-rubbery	As given for respiratory viruses Samples for BVDV testing: skin or EDTA blood; or mucosal erosions, Peyer patch, spleen, lymph node

Dictyocaulus viviparus: acute prepatent disease as a result of larval migration, or chronic patent or postpatent infection	Acute: lungs are diffusely red, edematous, and firm (interstitial pneumonia) Chronic: adult worms in caudal bronchi (see **Fig. 1H**), lobular atelectasis, or consolidation of lung tissue, especially in *dorsocaudal* areas of lung	Acute: histopathology to identify larvae/immature parasites in lung. Chronic: gross finding of worms in bronchi; histopathologic examination as given Live animals: Baermann test to identify larvae in chilled feces, but not in prepatent or postpatent infections Serologic tests may be useful for herd diagnosis[16]
Ascaris suum larval migration	Generalized distribution of lobular atelectasis or consolidation	Histopathologic examination to identify larvae in lung Eggs or larvae are NOT present in feces
Heart disease causing pulmonary edema	Diffusely red-purple heavy lungs, interlobular edema, ooze fluid from the cut surface, abundant foam or fluid in trachea	Clinical, gross, or histologic evidence of heart disease
Anaphylaxis causing pulmonary edema and bronchoconstriction	Diffusely red-purple heavy lungs, interlobular edema, ooze fluid from the cut surface, abundant foam or fluid in trachea	Clinical history; rule out cardiac causes of edema; histopathology shows edema ± eosinophils depending on the timing
Tuberculosis (*M bovis*)	Single or multiple soft white raised granulomas, often with caseous necrosis and/or mineralization in the center	Histopathology and acid-fast stain ± special culture procedure Similar gross lesions can represent bacterial or fungal pyogranulomas, chronic abscesses, or hydatid cysts[17]
Ingested toxins: L-tryptophan/3-methylindole (lush forage), 4-ipomeanol (moldy sweet potatoes), perilla ketone (purple mint)	Lungs are diffusely edematous and firm (interstitial pneumonia, see **Fig. 1C**)	Histopathologic examination confirms interstitial lung injury Diagnosis is based on clinical findings and identification of the source of toxin
Inhaled toxins: silo or pit gas, etc	As given	As given
Hypersensitivity pneumonitis	Diffusely firm and heavy lungs	Histopathologic and clinical findings
Contagious bovine pleuropneumonia (*Mycoplasma mycoides* ssp *mycoides* SC)	Often unilateral, caudal lung lobe consolidation with sequestrum formation, and fibrinous pleuritis	Culture of nasal swabs, pleural exudate, lung, lymph node Reportable OIE List A disease

(*continued on next page*)

Table 1
(continued)

Cause	Gross Lesions	Laboratory Diagnosis
Tracheal edema and hemorrhage ("honker") syndrome	Tracheal mucosa is thickened by edema and hemorrhage, obstructing the lumen	Gross findings
Pulmonary emphysema, secondary to nonpulmonary disease	Interlobular septa distended by air bubbles, especially in dorsocaudal lung, with normal texture of lung lobules	Gross findings

Abbreviations: BCV, bovine coronavirus; BHV, bovine herpesvirus 1; BPI3V, bovine parainfluenza virus 3; BRSV, bovine respiratory syncytial virus; BVDV, bovine viral diarrhea virus; ELISA, enzyme-linked immunosorbent assay; IHC, immunohistochemistry; OIE, world organization for animal health; PCR, polymerase chain reaction; PI, persistently infected; RT, reverse transcriptase; VI, virus isolation.

[a] Tests performed on fixed tissues: histopathology and IHC (for test availability, see http://ihc.sdstate.org/). With the exception of BVDV IHC for detection of PI animals, IHC is rarely a stand-alone test. The decision to pursue IHC testing is typically based on histologic lesions present, and results are interpreted in the context of these lesions.

[b] Tests performed on chilled or frozen tissues: VI, PCR, RT-PCR, and antigen-capture ELISA and other immunoassays.

Table 2
Diagnostic approaches to determine the cause of an outbreak of BRD

Diagnostic Approach	Advantages	Disadvantages
Detect an agent in clinical samples: nasal or nasopharyngeal swabs, transtracheal wash, bronchoalveolar lavage.	Rapid test results are possible. Multiple animals may be sampled, cases and controls. Identification of a virus may be highly significant, depending on the nature of the herd.	Viral infections are transient. Identification is impaired by rising antibody titers. Bacterial isolates from nasal samples are of dubious significance.
Serology to detect rising antibody titers	High sensitivity: most respiratory pathogens of cattle induce a strong antibody response. Less time-dependent than other methods, and may be effective even relatively late in the course of disease. Multiple animals tested makes the result relevant to the herd problem.	Requires convalescent serum, so results are not available for >3 wk. Testing of multiple samples can be expensive. Correlation of seroconversion with clinical disease may be impossible in situations when viral infections are expected to be common, such as recently arrived feedlot cattle.
Postmortem examination with subsequent laboratory testing	Gross and histopathologic examination usually suggests a cause and may be pathognomonic. The investigation is comprehensive and robust and leads to diseases that were not previously considered or recognized. Lung and trachea are easily sampled and are often the ideal samples for laboratory diagnosis.	Diagnosis may be based on few animals. Animals that die may not be representative of the herd problem. Death may occur at a subacute stage of disease, when viral pathogens are no longer present. Cases are often treated with antibiotics before death, precluding isolation of bacterial pathogens and resulting in misleading antimicrobial sensitivity data.

Box 1
Gross pathologic examination in cases of respiratory disease

A. Lesions in other body systems

Postmortem examination in cases of respiratory disease must not only focus on the respiratory system but also search for clues in other body systems.

- Bovine viral diarrhea virus (BVDV) is an important predisposing cause of bacterial pneumonia, so oral and esophageal erosions and Peyer patch necrosis should be actively sought at necropsy. However, many BVDV-infected calves have no gross lesions.

- Heart disease causes pulmonary edema with dyspnea and hyperpnea, and the prosector should search for abscesses or infarcts in the left ventricular papillary muscle caused by *Histophilus somni,* for bacterial endocarditis of the valves, and for congenital anomalies.

- Heart lesions may not be detected grossly and the diagnosis may depend on histologic evidence of myocarditis caused by BVDV or on myocardial necrosis resulting from toxin exposure or white muscle disease. In cases of respiratory distress in which a reliable diagnosis is not achieved by gross necropsy examination, formalin-fixed samples of heart (and other tissues) should always be included in the diagnostic investigation. For example, we recognize a fatal condition in feedlot cattle with mild bronchopneumonia as the only gross lesion, but lymphocytic necrotizing arteritis attributed to BVDV infection is obvious if multiple sections of lung, heart, and other organs are examined histologically.

- When opening the pulmonic valve, continue the incision to open the main branches of the pulmonary arteries. Pulmonary emboli—a cause of either peracute or chronic disease—are routinely overlooked if this important step is neglected (see **Fig. 1**F).

B. Examination of the upper airways

- The pluck—tongue, larynx, esophagus, trachea, lungs, and heart—should be removed at the time of necropsy. If the lungs are only examined in situ, unilateral lesions will be overlooked, and it is unlikely that the upper respiratory tract and heart will be effectively examined. Evaluation of the nasal cavity requires sectioning with a saw or axe. Examination of the upper respiratory tract may reveal miscellaneous causes of inspiratory dyspnea, including laryngeal lesions of diphtheria, focal masses obstructing airflow, or cellulitis of the head or neck.

- In infectious bovine rhinotracheitis (IBR), the primary viral infection typically causes nonfatal febrile illness with respiratory distress; fatalities generally result from secondary bacterial bronchopneumonia. Lesions of tracheal erosion are essentially pathognomonic of IBR. In cases of bacterial bronchopneumonia, expectorated mucus, pus, or fibrin covers the tracheal mucosa and can easily be mistaken for lesions of IBR. However, this material is easily wiped from the tracheal mucosa, revealing a smooth intact mucosa, whereas cases of IBR have adherent exudate or multifocal pale areas of mucosal necrosis. Nevertheless, in autolyzed cases, this distinction can be problematic.

- Examination of the large airways should not end at the tracheal bifurcation and must persevere to the bronchi in the caudal lung. Adult *Dictyocaulus* worms preferentially reside in these caudal bronchi (see **Fig. 1**H), and finding these worms provides an immediate and high-impact diagnosis that may forestall hundreds of dollars of laboratory testing.

C. Examination of the lungs

In many cases, the lungs hold the important clues that direct subsequent investigation, but some misleading changes must be recognized.

- Red discoloration of lung tissue commonly results from postmortem pooling of blood as veins dilate after death. Visible reddening indicates specific areas of the lung that should be carefully palpated and perhaps sampled histologically. However, diffuse or patchy red discoloration throughout the lung is usually a postmortem artifact, and localized discoloration with no change in texture should be interpreted with much caution. The dorsocaudal lung of cattle is normally white and opaque because the pleura in this area is thick and fibrous, but this must not be mistaken for an abnormality (see **Fig. 1**C, E). Interlobular and subpleural emphysema, appearing as lines of air-filled bubbles separating the lobules, arises commonly in cattle that are dyspneic for any reason (see **Fig. 1C, D**). Pulmonary emphysema occurs without other lung disease, for example in downer cows dying of toxic mastitis or hypocalcemia, but it is a clue to look for more diagnostically specific lesions such as firmness of the individual lung lobules that separate the emphysematous interlobular septa.

- Palpation—the key to effective examination of the lung—must be based on a *cut section* of lung because the thick pleura is a barrier to effective palpation. Superficial palpation is useless, and the fingers must push deeply, like microscopic probes assessing the texture of each individual lobule. It is useful to categorize the abnormal lung texture on a 5-point scale that often correlates with the morphologic pattern of lung disease:

  - Hard and crisp, as a result of peracute fibrinous bronchopneumonia

  - Firm or liver-like, as a result of acute or chronic bronchopneumonia

  - Slightly firm or rubbery, as a result of bronchointerstitial or interstitial pneumonia

  - Wet and heavy, but of essentially normal texture, as a result of edema

  - Spongier than normal, as a result of air trapping from airway obstruction or emphysema

- The distribution and the texture of the lung lesions are the basis for identifying the morphologic pattern of disease (see **Table 3**).

bronchopneumonia typical of infection with Pasteurellaceae bacteria. There were multinucleated cells in alveoli, but these were more likely macrophage giant cells instead of the epithelial syncytia seen in BRSV infection. A single bronchiolar epithelial cell seemed to have a cytoplasmic inclusion body, suggestive of BRSV or BPI3V, but this was not considered conclusive.

Pathologists and practitioners sometimes find such suggestive but non-diagnostic lesions to be disappointing. Nevertheless, these findings are indispensible in 2 ways:

- When laboratory testing identifies a pathogen, the presence of a compatible histologic lesion provides considerable confidence that the pathogen is indeed causing disease in that animal.
- Histopathologic changes often indicate the disease process and the likely types of pathogens responsible, even if better samples, other animals, or more appropriate assays are required to identify the pathogen.

In addition to formalin-fixed tissue, lung samples from this case had been individually bagged, chilled on freezer packs, and transported overnight to the laboratory. Available tests and preferred diagnostic methods vary considerably between diagnostic laboratories, so test selection must be based on the user's guide for each laboratory or consultation with laboratory personnel. In this case, results of initial testing of lung samples were:

- Immunohistochemistry: negative for BRSV and BHV-1
- Bacterial culture: no pathogens identified
- Fluorescent antibody test: negative for BPI3V, BRSV, and BHV-1

These results raise a consideration of the reasons for discrepant or unexpectedly negative test results. General considerations are outlined in **Box 4**. Histologic findings in this case of bronchointerstitial pneumonia fit well with the clinical picture of viral pneumonia and motivated further investigation of the cause. Subsequently, immunohistochemical testing for BVDV, BCV, and BPI3V was performed: BVDV infection does

Table 3
Morphologic patterns of lung disease

Morphologic Pattern	Typical Gross Lesions: Distribution and Texture	Major Causes
1. Bronchopneumonia		
1a. Bilateral	Cranioventral distribution, more or less bilaterally symmetric, hard and crisp or firm and liver-like (see **Fig. 1A**).	Opportunistic bacteria, usually Pasteurellaceae
1b. Asymmetric or focal	Usually cranial or middle lung lobes, focal or asymmetrical. Often necrotic, putrid, and green-brown	Aspiration of rumen content, feed, or administered substances
2. Interstitial and bronchointerstitial pneumonia[a]		
2a. Generalized interstitial lung injury	Diffuse or lobular ("checkerboard") lesions, generalized to all lung lobes (see **Fig. 1C**). Subtle firmness or rubbery texture, with alveolar and interlobular edema. Lesions may be obscured by interlobular emphysema.	Respiratory viruses, septicemia, endotoxemia, parasitic larval migration, idiopathic interstitial pneumonia of feedlot cattle, toxic lung disease, hypersensitivity pneumonitis
2b. Cranioventral bronchointerstitial pneumonia	Cranioventral lung has slightly firm-rubbery texture, collapse, and reddening (see **Fig. 1D**). Dorsocaudal lung is heavy and edematous, often with interlobular emphysema.	Respiratory viruses, such as BRSV. Note that these viruses may also cause generalized interstitial lung injury.
2c. Generalized interstitial lung injury plus cranioventral bronchopneumonia	Dorsocaudal regions are slightly firm-rubbery, like for generalized interstitial lung injury, but cranioventral areas are consolidated as a result of bacterial bronchopneumonia.	Viral pneumonia with secondary bacterial pneumonia. Idiopathic, perhaps acute lung injury secondary to bacterial pneumonia
3. Embolic lung lesions		
3a. Multifocal embolic pneumonia	Multifocal lesions in all lobes (see **Fig. 1E**). Firm consolidation or abscesses	Embolism or bacteremia from heart, liver, caudal vena cava, jugular veins, and uterus
3b. Thromboembolism	Thrombi occluding large branches of the pulmonary arteries (see **Fig. 1F**)	Embolism, as given
4. Pleuritis		
	Exudate on pleural surface, with or without consolidation of underlying lung tissue (see **Fig. 1G**)	H somni pleuritis, pleuropneumonia as a result of Pasteurellaceae bacteria, penetrating injury, Escherichia coli bacteremia in young calves, or ruptured abscess

[a] The various gross appearances of interstitial/bronchointerstitial pneumonia may cause confusion. The term is based on the histologic appearance of the lesions, which remains constant whether the gross lesions are generalized, cranioventral, or complicated by bronchopneumonia.

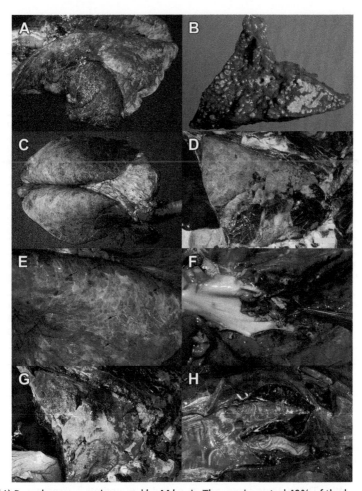

Fig. 1. (*A*) Bronchopneumonia caused by M bovis. The cranioventral 40% of the lung is brick red and consolidated and contains innumerable pale, round approximately 3-mm-diameter nodules. Left lung: trachea is to the left. (*B*) M bovis bronchopneumonia. Section of lung with multiple coalescing nodules of caseous necrosis. (*C*) Generalized interstitial lung injury. The lung fails to collapse, is heavy as a result of edema, and has a generalized firm-rubbery texture. Interlobular septa contain innumerable tiny air bubbles (interlobular emphysema). A specific cause was not identified. Note the white opacity of the dorsocaudal pleura, which is normal in bovine lung. (*D*) Cranioventral bronchointerstitial pneumonia caused by BRSV. The cranioventral (lower right) 25% of the lung is collapsed and plum red and has a slightly firm-rubbery texture (but lacks the more obvious liver-like firmness that would be typical of bronchopneumonia). The dorsocaudal lung has a similar texture, with extensive interlobular emphysema. Right lung: trachea is to the right. (*E*) Embolic pneumonia. All lung lobes are peppered by 2- to 10-mm-diameter raised firm purple-red nodules (arrows), which had purulent exudate on cut section. The source of the infection was septic cellulitis and venous thrombosis, as a complication of a toggle surgery for displaced abomasum. Left lung: trachea is to the left. (*F*) Pulmonary embolism secondary to endocarditis. A ragged embolism fills the opened pulmonary artery. This lesion is easily overlooked if the arteries are not opened. Dorsal view of left lung: heart is to the left and caudal lung is to the right. (*G*) Fibrinous pleuritis caused by Histophilus somni. Yellow-white fibrin and fluid cover the pleural surface of the lung. The lung tissue is congested and edematous, but otherwise normal. Right lung: trachea is to the right. (*H*) Dictyocaulus viviparus. The caudal bronchi contain frothy fluid with a few adult nematodes. Dorsal view: trachea is to the left. Normal pink lobules contrasted with purple-red consolidated ones, in the adjacent lung tissue. ([*G*] Courtesy of Dr Heindrich N. Snyman.)

Table 4
Differentiating clinical and epidemiologic features of BRD that are of most importance to laboratory diagnosticians[a]

Clinical Features	Possible Interpretation or Cause
Basic epidemiologic information: time since arrival at a new facility or introduction of new animals, number at risk, proportion affected, case fatality rate and characteristics, age range of affected calves, attributes of affected and unaffected cattle, and duration of the disease.	
Outbreak or endemic disease	Viruses, parasites, and toxins are major considerations for outbreaks.
Pasture or housed	*Dictyocaulus* worms cause disease in pastured or formerly pastured animals. 3-Methylindole toxicity is associated with recent access to lush pasture.
Fever	Bacterial, viral, acute parasitism
Severity of depression relative to severity of dyspnea	Severe depression suggests bacterial pneumonia. Severe dyspnea suggests viral or parasitic pneumonia.
Inspiratory or expiratory dyspnea	Inspiratory dyspnea or stridor suggests upper respiratory tract obstruction, whereas expiratory dyspnea suggests pulmonary or cardiac disease.
Lameness	*M bovis, H somni*
Response to antibiotic therapy, vaccination history	Implications with respect to bacterial or viral infections

[a] This key information should be included with the diagnostic submission.

not cause primary lung disease but is an important predisposing cause of bacterial pneumonia and should be considered in any herd problem of respiratory disease, whereas BCV is an uncommon but underrecognized cause of viral pneumonia in cattle. These tests were negative, but a quantitative ("real-time") reverse

Box 2
Selection of animals for sampling

- Examine multiple animals.

- Animals should be selected that are representative of the disease problem with respect to clinical signs, age, and pen grouping. Ensure that the expensive investigation is not conducted on those that have died of other causes.

- Examine early in disease course, at the onset of clinical signs. Experimental studies suggest that animals in the first 1–4 days of clinical illness are most likely to shed virus (with virus detectable at 4–7 days after infection for bovine respiratory syncytial virus [BRSV] and other viruses).[18–20] An absence of fever suggests that the animal is not likely to have active respiratory viral infection, but the converse is not true: animals may remain febrile after the pathogen has been cleared, for example, if there is secondary bacterial pneumonia. Serum haptoglobin and other acute phase proteins (APPs) remain elevated throughout the duration of the inflammatory response and thus do not necessarily indicate *acute* disease. Using APPs to select affected animals for testing is also currently constrained by the delay needed for laboratory testing.

- Examine animals that were not treated with antibiotics, if identification of bacterial pathogens and their antimicrobial susceptibility is desirable.

Box 3
Tissue sampling at necropsy

Selection of tissue samples

- Unless there is considerable confidence in the diagnosis at the time of necropsy, it is recommended to submit *nonrespiratory tissues* as part of the respiratory disease investigation. Examples of significant microscopic lesions in nonrespiratory tissues include myocardial lesions causing heart failure and dyspnea, lymphocytic arteritis in the heart or depletion of lymphoid tissue as a result of BVDV infection, intestinal lesions as a result of bovine coronavirus (BCV) or BVDV, and various inflammatory lesions as the basis for febrile illnesses that may mimic bacterial pneumonia.

- *Upper respiratory tract* samples should be taken: nasal cavity, larynx, and trachea.

  o Nasal swabs are effective for identification of respiratory viruses, including BRSV, bovine parainfluenza virus-1 (BPI3V), bovine herpesvirus-1 (BHV-1), and BCV.

  o Bacteria isolated from nasal swabs are not well correlated with those from the lung, although there is some controversy in the literature on this point: isolates are the same species only 68% of the time and may be present in nasal swabs without causing disease, yet antimicrobial sensitivity of isolates seem to be similar in both locations.[21–23]

- Sampling of lung tissue

  o Histopathology and immunohistochemistry: Sample at least 3–5 areas, including samples from the border between abnormal and normal lung and a sample from normal lung. Samples must cover the spectrum of lesions in the lung; for example, a single lung may have cranioventral consolidation, abscesses, dorsocaudal interstitial pneumonia, and pleuritis, and all should be examined histologically.

  o Virology: Take 2 samples from the cranioventral lung and 1 from the dorsocaudal lung. Viral antigen and nucleic acid are of nonuniform distribution, and some cases have BRSV in the cranioventral but not the caudodorsal lung.[24,25]

  o Bacterial culture: Sample consolidated lung tissue near the border between abnormal and normal lung, avoiding abscesses. Bacterial pathogens are most reliably detected in consolidated lung tissue near the junction with normal lung. This represents the anatomic site that has most recently become infected, whereas the older lesions in the cranioventral area are more likely to be colonized by secondary pathogens. Samples of lung tissue should be ≥4 cm in diameter. Compared with swabs taken in the field, contamination of lung tissue samples may be less likely if a tissue block is submitted, because the surface is seared in the laboratory before sampling for culture. Conversely, swabs have the advantage of ease of use and improved preservation during transport.

  o *M bovis*: Foci of caseous necrosis are ideal, or areas of consolidation.

  o Tuberculosis: Caseating granulomas in lung (usually a single granuloma), in mediastinal, tracheabronchial, and retropharyngeal lymph nodes, and palatine tonsils.[17]

- Tissue preservation

  o Samples for histopathology and immunohistochemistry are fixed in formalin. Small pieces, 1 cm thick, are ideal, with a 1:10 ratio of tissue to formalin. Large blocks of tissue autolyze during transport, because formalin does not penetrate to the center of the sample.

  o Samples for bacterial culture, virus isolation, and molecular testing are chilled with freezer packs or refrigerated. Frozen samples are also useful, especially when tissues are held pending the outcome of initial tests.

  o Swabs for bacterial culture or virus isolation are preserved in bacterial or viral transport medium, respectively, and chilled. The success of virus isolation is much reduced for swabs preserved in bacterial transport medium.

Box 4
Interpretation of negative diagnostic laboratory data

When laboratory tests to detect an antigen, nucleic acid, culturable pathogen, or antibody unexpectedly fail, general considerations include the following:

A. *Incorrect clinical diagnosis*: The suspected pathogen is not the cause, and alternative possibilities should be considered.

B. *Disease without active infection*: The pathogen is the cause of the disease, but it is no longer present in the animal.

- BRSV and BPI3V are difficult to detect after 7–8 days postinfection, corresponding to a few days of clinical signs.[18–20] In these cases, submitting samples from more acutely infected animals or measuring titers in acute and convalescent samples is a pathway to a definitive diagnosis.

- Bacteria may be eliminated or fail to grow in culture as a result of antibiotic treatment.

- *Dictyocaulus*: During the acute phase of larval migration through the lung (7–25 days after infection), adults are not yet present in bronchi nor are there larvae in feces. Conversely, chronic or postpatent infections can still elicit clinical signs, despite the absence of adult worms in the lung or larvae in the feces. Finally, partially immune animals that are reinfected can develop severe disease, yet the infection never becomes patent. The results of the Baermann test on feces are negative in all 3 of these situations: acute prepatent, postpatent, and partially immune nonpatent infections.

C. *Inadequate samples:* The pathogen is the cause of the disease, but the samples are inadequate. See sampling strategies in **Boxes 2** and **3**.

- BRSV has a generalized distribution in the lung in some cases but is present only in the cranioventral lung in others.[24,25] Samples for virology testing should include 3 samples, including both the cranial and the caudal lung.

- Sampling from abscesses instead of actively infected tissue is likely to yield secondary pathogens.

- Sample autolysis as a result of inappropriate storage or transport of chilled specimens results in degradation of antigens and loss of viability of culturable pathogens. Immunohistochemical tests fail if tissues are autolyzed or underfixed, if the volume of formalin is too small, or if excessively large samples of tissue are used (1-cm-thick pieces are adequate for histopathologic examination).

- Freeze-thaw cycles are harmful, and they may occur from storage of samples in frost-free freezers or from thawing during transport.

- Prolonged fixation may interfere with antigen detection by immunohistochemistry: fixing for <1 week is generally recommended, although improved methods allow antigen retrieval with up to 7 weeks of fixation.[26] Bouin solution or other alternatives to formalin fixation may affect immunohistochemical detection of some antigens,[27,28] but the addition of ethanol to prevent freezing (to a final concentration of 10%) is considered safe.

D. *Test failure:* The pathogen is present in the sample but was not detected.

- Antibody interference: Antibody in the diagnostic specimen interferes with the ability of the test to detect the pathogen. The antibody may result from colostral transfer of maternal antibody, from vaccination, or from development of an immune response following infection. Such antibody may not protect against disease, yet may interfere with the ability of an immunoassay to detect viral antigen (eg, antigen-capture enzyme-linked immunosorbent assay) or inhibit growth of virus in tissue culture (virus isolation).

- "Inhibitors" are substances in the sample that interfere with molecular detection of pathogens. This problem should be detected by routine quality control procedures in the laboratory.

- It is possible that genetic variants are not detected by routine diagnostic tests, particularly for RNA viruses. Although assays are tested during development against a broad collection of archived and contemporary isolates, it is possible that emerging strains of a pathogen are not detected by current tests.[29]

- Practitioners are dependent on a quality assurance program in the diagnostic laboratory, including test validation, appropriate use of positive and negative control samples, and valid interpretation of test data. Test results that conflict with clinical findings might represent laboratory error, and discussion with laboratory personnel can occasionally be fruitful in these circumstances.

transcriptase–polymerase chain reaction (RT-PCR) test for BRSV was performed subsequently and the results were positive.

Findings supporting the diagnosis of BRSV in this case were the clinical picture, the histologic diagnosis of bronchointerstitial pneumonia with a single equivocal inclusion body, and the quantitative RT-PCR result. These contrasted with the negative results of the immunohistochemistry and fluorescent antibody tests and the absence of histologically evident syncytia. Reasons for the discrepancy in this case are speculative. The animal may have been subacutely infected, with little viral antigen remaining in the lung. Test sensitivity is a likely contributor: immunohistochemistry has the advantage that the best histologic lesions are selected for testing, and the test results are easily interpreted in conjunction with the histologic findings, yet prior studies have identified that quantitative RT-PCR testing for BRSV is more sensitive than other available tests.[15,24,30] Further, because the 2 tests in this case were performed on different pieces of tissue, uneven distribution of antigen may have randomly resulted in one test being positive and the other negative. Laboratory quality control and overfixation of tissues were not thought to contribute to the negative tests in this case, based on appropriate results in control samples. The failure to detect bacterial pathogens despite histologic evidence of bronchopneumonia was presumed to have resulted from antibiotic treatment before death or perhaps from incorrect sample selection.

False-positive tests may also occur, and causes include laboratory error, contamination between specimens from different cases, and vaccination in the past 20 days.[31] For herpesvirus infections, stress- or glucocorticoid-induced reactivation of latent infection may be detected by diagnostic testing, even if the herpesvirus played no role in causing the clinical disease. Thus, when discrepancies occur, a positive test should not automatically be considered more reliable than a negative test.

This case illustrates the laboratory investigation of BRD using samples obtained at necropsy and followed a somewhat standardized protocol. The initial testing provided clues but was nondiagnostic and somewhat conflicting, and an inadequate laboratory submission may have ended with this unsatisfactory outcome. However, the accurate clinical history and the availability of lung samples permitted — and indeed motivated — the subsequent testing that led to the diagnosis. This illustrates a major virtue of the necropsy: the breadth of the examination and the variety of samples collected permit a comprehensive and robust diagnostic investigation that can be amended according to interim test results.

All calves in the pen were treated with antibiotics at the time the group was initially examined, and further deaths were not noted. BRSV was considered the cause of the outbreak and the producer was advised on prevention of future recurrences, but the herd remains unvaccinated.

CASE 2: ONGOING PROBLEMS WITH RESPIRATORY DISEASE IN A BEEF HERD

A small 30-head beef herd was examined in late October because of respiratory disease in 20 of the cows and calves. Half of the cases involved the mature animals. A cow and a bull had been purchased in September, and the herd was usually vaccinated and dewormed in the autumn but this had not yet been done this year. Clinical signs included fever, cough, hyperpnea, dyspnea, frothing at the mouth, and weight loss. A field necropsy of 3 animals revealed consolidation of the lungs, interpreted as bacterial bronchopneumonia.

A 4-year-old cow from the herd died after more than 2 weeks of weight loss and respiratory disease, which had been nonresponsive to sequential therapy with florfenicol, tilmicosin, and penicillin. The cow was submitted to the diagnostic laboratory, and necropsy revealed numerous lungworms and catarrhal exudate in bronchi of all lobes (see **Fig. 1**H for a different case, albeit with fewer worms). The cranial and middle lobes were reddened and consolidated, all lobes had multifocal 2- to 8-mm-diameter firm red-purple lesions, and interlobular emphysema was most prominent in the caudal lobes. *Klebsiella pneumoniae* was isolated in large number from both samples of lung tested. Histopathology did not reveal evidence of bronchopneumonia, but the nodular and consolidated lesions corresponded to pyogranulomatous inflammation centered on caseous foci containing aspirated eggs and larvae, and chronic parasitic bronchitis and bronchiolitis were present.

The diagnosis of lungworm was verified on one additional animal that died on the farm. Testing fecal samples from multiple animals, to detect larvae using the Baermann technique, would be an alternative method to establish the extent of infection in the group. This technique is highly sensitive and is reported to be capable of detecting a single egg-producing worm, at those stages when the infection is patent.[32] The herd problem was reported to have resolved quickly after treatment of the herd with ivermectin.

The case is notable because diagnoses of *Dictyocaulus* spp are uncommon in this herd's geographic area, as in many areas of North America. However, it does occur in most areas and is of particular diagnostic significance because the therapy and control strategies are so different from those of other BRDs. The case is an effective illustration of the value of a thorough necropsy examination, the ease with which diagnostically important lesions can be overlooked, and the importance of dogged persistence and examination of multiple animals in conducting a diagnostic investigation. The cause of a disease problem can usually be identified by a systematic, insightful, and tenacious herd-level investigation, even if the initial attempts have failed.

CASE 3: SEROLOGIC INVESTIGATION OF UPPER RESPIRATORY DISEASE IN A DAIRY HERD

A Holstein dairy herd with 40 milking cows experienced a respiratory disease outbreak in 20% of the cows. The herd had had no outside introductions for years, and artificial insemination was used. Annual vaccination with killed vaccines for BHV, BVDV, BPI3V and BRSV was last done 11 months previously. The facility was a bank barn, with milking cows in 2 rows of tie stalls. The producer noted significant amounts of blood and fibrin in the manger. Affected cows had obvious dyspnea, until they dislodged a fibrin plug from their nasal cavity, when they seemed more normal and would eat. Only 3 cows were treated with antibiotics, and none died.

Pens containing 8 young calves were adjacent to one of the rows of milking cows, and all of these had clinical signs of pneumonia that developed a few days after the disease outbreak in the cows. Calves were treated with antibiotics, and 1 died. Pens of older ($\sim$1 year of age) calves elsewhere in the same barn had no clinical signs.

This is an unusual clinical presentation, and a diagnosis was not immediately apparent. A field postmortem examination of the dead calf revealed fibrinous bronchopneumonia. Although laboratory testing of tissues from this animal might have been useful, it was uncertain whether the problem in the calves was the same as the more perplexing problem in the cows. Instead, the diagnostic investigation focused on the cows, in an effort to ensure that the results were applicable to the problem of most concern.

A diagnostic option, which was not pursued in this case, would have been to attempt to isolate a virus from nasal swabs or samples of the dislodged fibrin plugs.

With this method, identifying a viral pathogen would be of reliable significance in a closed herd with compatible clinical signs. However, because the practitioner was not involved at the onset of the outbreak in the cows and was only later called to the farm when the calves became ill, there would be a risk that active viral infection might no longer be detected.

Instead, the diagnostic quest in this case was based on serologic examination. Samples were collected at the time of the initial visit and 3 weeks later, from 5 affected cows and 5 of the affected young calves. Data are shown in **Table 5**.

Observations and interpretation of these data are as follows:

1. Four of the 5 cows tested had a greater than 4-fold increase in titers to BPI3V, in the convalescent compared to the acute serum samples. In a closed herd in which active parainfluenza virus infection is expected to be uncommon and in the presence of compatible clinical signs, the authors interpret this to be the cause of the outbreak. Others have described a comparable outbreak of upper respiratory disease characterized by fever, nasal discharge with erosions, and submandibular swelling in vaccinated adult cows that was associated with seroconversion to this virus.[33] The authors are not aware of any description of this condition in the peer-reviewed literature.
2. None of the calves seroconverted to BPI3V, confirming the just-noted suspicion that the disease in the calves differed from that in the cows.
3. There was a consistent trend of higher titers in young calves and lower titers in older calves, for all viruses tested except BRSV. This is interpreted to represent decay of maternal antibody as the calves age.
4. Titers to BRSV were considerably higher in older than in younger calves, but none seroconverted. We would not rule out the possibility that this virus caused the disease in the calves, but this remains uncertain.

The laboratory fees for measuring a single serum antibody titer are low compared with the costs of histopathologic examination, virus isolation, or molecular testing. However, it is of limited value and sometimes highly misleading to evaluate titers in single serum samples, so acute and convalescent sera from several animals are required to properly assess the relationship of seroconversion with disease. The total cost of such a diagnostic investigation can be startling.

This case illustrates the value of serologic investigation as a reliable method of establishing a diagnosis, even some time after the beginning of the outbreak. None of the veterinarians were aware that BPI3V could cause this form of respiratory disease, and an unusual manifestation of IBR was considered likely at the time. A well-planned diagnostic investigation allowed the authors to stumble upon diagnoses of which they were not aware. This presents a notable contrast with case 1, in which the clinical findings suggestive of respiratory disease served to direct the laboratory investigation.

CASE 4: LABORATORY TESTING TO IDENTIFY CATTLE WITH RESPIRATORY DISEASE

Tromping through a beef feedlot in Alberta were the experienced operator of the large Western feedlot and a veterinary pathologist and a veterinary student from small-farm Ontario. For each calf in the pen, questions were raised: Is it sick? Does it have bacterial pneumonia? Is it affected severely enough to require antibiotic treatment? One calf was obviously sick and later determined to have a fever. But another calf had been under observation by the producer since the previous day, with a subtle tendency to stay apart from its mates and away from the feed bunk. The authors decided,

Table 5
Serology data from an outbreak of upper respiratory disease in a dairy herd

	BAV	BCV	BRSV	BVDV	BHV-1	BPI3V
Cow 1	3	256	3072	32	48	1536
	3	**256**	**2048**	**24**	**48**	**>4096**
Cow 2	48	256	4096	768	48	1536
	48	**512**	**4096**	**768**	**48**	**4096**
Cow 3	3	512	3072	4	6	768
	2	**512**	**2048**	**2**	**12**	**>4096**
Cow 4	2	512	1536	384	16	1024
	3	**512**	**1536**	**256**	**32**	**>4096**
Cow 5	32	32	2048	256	32	1024
	24	**24**	**3072**	**256**	**64**	**>4096**
Calf 1 (oldest)	4	32	2048	12	<2	96
	3	**32**	**2048**	**6**	**<2**	**96**
Calf 2	<2	32	2048	6	2	64
	<2	**32**	**2048**	**6**	**2**	**96**
Calf 3	4	128	768	<2	2	384
	2	**128**	**512**	**<2**	**2**	**128**
Calf 4	24	128	384	128	32	512
	16	**128**	**384**	**96**	**16**	**768**
Calf 5 (youngest)	24	2048	1024	32	12	3072
	12	**2048**	**768**	**16**	**16**	**1024**

Data are the antibody titers in serum samples, for acute (upper rows) and convalescent (lower rows, bold font) samples, reported as the mean of the reciprocal log titers measured in duplicate.
Abbreviation: BAV, bovine adenovirus.

with considerable debate and uncertainty, that it was just homesick, and the decision was perhaps justified because it never did require antibiotic therapy.

Clinical examination from a distance—the art of pen checking—is an efficient screening test for disease in all production systems from large pens of beef steers to small groups of pastured dairy heifers, and most animals that require therapy to prevent death or chronic disease are identified with this method. However, even well-trained and experienced producers, staff, or veterinarians are imperfect and uncertain when it comes to distinguishing calves with disease from those experiencing distress as a result of recent weaning, transportation, processing, and disruption of social groups. Further distinction between respiratory disease and diseases of other body systems and between antibiotic-responsive pneumonia and nonbacterial causes of respiratory disease are even more imprecise based on clinical features alone. In a study to assess diagnosis of BRD by feedlot personnel, the sensitivity of BRD diagnosis by pen checkers was 94% and specificity was 77%.[34] Similarly, there was poor correlation between pulling a calf for suspected BRD and the presence of lung lesions at slaughter.[35] Further, these challenges only cover the need to identify those calves with severe bacterial pneumonia that without treatment would die or

---

Box 5
Laboratory tests to detect subclinical disease and to refine the clinical diagnosis

- Total white blood cell count and differential cell count are poor predictors of respiratory disease in feedlot cattle and do not significantly differentiate clinically sick from clinically normal animals in the first week after arrival. Similarly, these parameters, when measured in acutely sick calves, were not useful predictors of the severity of lung lesions at necropsy.[42,43]

- Arterial blood gas analysis and blood lactate levels do not reliably predict disease in challenged calves with mild lung lesions.[42] However, in cattle with severe respiratory disease, a plasma lactate concentration of 4 mmol/L predicted death within 24 hours.[44]

- Serum haptoglobin concentrations in serum or plasma increase following experimental *Mannheimia haemolytica* challenge of BHV-1–infected calves, and the degree of haptoglobin elevation correlated with disease severity, treatment failure, and greater likelihood of death.[45–47] Compared with the rapid (24 hours) increase in serum haptoglobin within 24 hours of the induction of pneumonic pasteurellosis, the response to BRSV or BVDV infection is more delayed, occurring during a period of 4–8 days and corresponding with the onset of a febrile response to the viral infection.[45,48–50] The findings of these experimental studies extend to the naturally occurring disease, in which increased serum haptoglobin level has been correlated with the presence of fever and clinical diagnosis of BRD.[46,47,51,52]

- Tests to measure other APPs, including lipopolysaccharide-binding protein and serum amyloid A, are not routinely available but may have advantages of earlier peak concentration.[50,53] In other studies, measuring fibrinogen, serum amyloid A, or α_1-acid glycoprotein, have not effectively distinguished between healthy cattle and those with respiratory disease under field conditions.[46,47,51,52]

- Animals need to be sampled early in the course of disease, at the onset of clinical signs, for haptoglobin and other APPs to have good diagnostic sensitivity and specificity. The sensitivity and specificity of detecting BRD are further improved by testing multiple APPs in parallel instead of using a single protein.[47] A peril in using APPs to detect BRD is that an increase in APPs reflects inflammation that is not specific to the respiratory system. Haptoglobin values were elevated to a similar degree as with BRD-affected calves when measured in dairy calves affected by diarrhea, umbilical infections, and oral abscesses.[51] Thus, a clinical assessment of the animal assists in the interpretation of elevated APP concentrations.

progress to chronic disease: it is likely that early treatment of more mildly affected calves would have a beneficial effect on retreatment rates, feed efficiency, growth, and carcass quality, but our ability to accurately identify these calves is limited.[36–39] In this scenario, if experienced feedlot operators and veterinarians are imprecise in making these determinations, what can the laboratory diagnostician from Ontario contribute?

Laboratory analysis of clinical samples can be a highly effective means of refining the clinical diagnosis in situations where the benefits of diagnosis outweigh the costs of acquiring and analyzing blood, nasal fluid, transtracheal wash, bronchoalveolar lavage, exhaled breath condensate, or lung biopsy samples.[40,41] **Box 5** outlines the methods and uses of laboratory analysis in this context.

SUMMARY

Pathologic and laboratory investigations are necessary in situations in which a specific diagnosis or identification of the cause is required. The 4 cases presented outline different approaches to laboratory diagnosis, including the microbiological analysis of samples obtained from animals that have died, the postmortem examination as a method of specific diagnosis, the investigation of a clinical mystery using serologic examination, and the use of laboratory testing to identify subclinical disease or refine the clinical diagnosis.

Elements of each diagnostic approach may hold merit in evaluating respiratory disease in cattle, and the diagnostic path will vary depending on the goals of the producer and veterinarian. Underscoring all approaches is the need to consider the herd history and evolution of clinical disease when trying to align clinical findings with the results of clinicopathologic, necropsy, and microbiologic testing. Open and ongoing discussion with the laboratory is key to optimizing test selection and interpretation.

ACKNOWLEDGMENTS

Dr Dave Douglas, Navan Veterinary Services; Dr Craig DeGroot, Tavistock Veterinary Service; Drs Susy Carman, Jan Shapiro, Beverly McEwen, Murray Hazlett. and Hugh Cai, Animal Health Laboratory, University of Guelph; and Drs David Sandals and Andrew Peregrine, Ontario Veterinary College, University of Guelph made considerable contributions to these cases and the article.

REFERENCES

1. Saif LJ. Bovine respiratory coronavirus. Vet Clin North Am Food Anim Pract 2010; 26(2):349–64.
2. Ellis JA. Bovine parainfluenza-3 virus. Vet Clin North Am Food Anim Pract 2010; 26(3):575–93.
3. Ridpath JF. The contribution of infections with bovine viral diarrhea viruses to bovine respiratory disease. Vet Clin North Am Food Anim Pract 2010;26(2): 335–48.
4. Griffin D. Bovine pasteurellosis and other bacterial infections of the respiratory tract. Vet Clin North Am Food Anim Pract 2010;26(1):57–71.
5. Brodersen BW. Bovine respiratory syncytial virus. Vet Clin North Am Food Anim Pract 2010;26(2):323–33.
6. Doster AR. Bovine atypical interstitial pneumonia. Vet Clin North Am Food Anim Pract 2010;26(2):395–407.

7. Bleul U. Respiratory distress syndrome in calves. Vet Clin North Am Food Anim Pract 2009;25(1):179–93.
8. Poulsen KP, McGuirk SM. Respiratory disease of the bovine neonate. Vet Clin North Am Food Anim Pract 2009;25(1):121–37.
9. Panciera RJ, Confer AW. Pathogenesis and pathology of bovine pneumonia. Vet Clin North Am Food Anim Pract 2010;26(2):191–214.
10. Caswell JL, Williams K. The respiratory system. In: Maxie M, editor. Pathology of domestic animals, vol. 2, 5th edition. New York: Saunders; 2007. p. 523–653.
11. Cooper VL, Brodersen BW. Respiratory disease diagnostics of cattle. Vet Clin North Am Food Anim Pract 2010;26(2):409–16.
12. Nietfeld JC. Field necropsy techniques and proper specimen submission for investigation of emerging infectious diseases of food animals. Vet Clin North Am Food Anim Pract 2010;26(1):1–13.
13. Apley M. Antimicrobials and BRD. Anim Health Res Rev 2009;10(2):159–61.
14. Lamm CG, Love BC, Krehbiel CR, et al. Comparison of antemortem antimicrobial treatment regimens to antimicrobial susceptibility patterns of postmortem lung isolates from feedlot cattle with bronchopneumonia. J Vet Diagn Invest 2012; 24(2):277–82. http://dx.doi.org/10.1177/1040638711428149.
15. Timsit E, Maingourd C, Dréan EL, et al. Evaluation of a commercial real-time reverse transcription polymerase chain reaction kit for the diagnosis of bovine respiratory syncytial virus infection. J Vet Diagn Invest 2010;22(2):238–41.
16. Klewer A, Forbes A, Schnieder T, et al. A survey on Dictyocaulus viviparus antibodies in bulk milk of dairy herds in northern Germany. Prev Vet Med 2012; 103(2–3):243–5.
17. Liebana E, Johnson L, Gough J, et al. Pathology of naturally occurring bovine tuberculosis in England and Wales. Vet J 2008;176(3):354–60.
18. Bryson DG, McNulty MS, Logan EF, et al. Respiratory syncytial virus pneumonia in young calves: clinical and pathologic findings. Am J Vet Res 1983;44(9):1648–55.
19. McNulty MS, Bryson DG, Allan GM. Experimental respiratory syncytial virus pneumonia in young calves: microbiologic and immunofluorescent findings. Am J Vet Res 1983;44(9):1656–9.
20. Castleman WL, Lay JC, Dubovi EJ, et al. Experimental bovine respiratory syncytial virus infection in conventional calves: light microscopic lesions, microbiology, and studies on lavaged lung cells. Am J Vet Res 1985;46(3):547–53.
21. Allen JW, Viel L, Bateman KG, et al. The microbial flora of the respiratory tract in feedlot calves: associations between nasopharyngeal and bronchoalveolar lavage cultures. Can J Vet Res 1991;55(4):341–6.
22. DeRosa DC, Mechor GD, Staats JJ, et al. Comparison of Pasteurella spp. simultaneously isolated from nasal and transtracheal swabs from cattle with clinical signs of bovine respiratory disease. J Clin Microbiol 2000;38(1): 327–32.
23. Sheehan M, Markey B, Cassidy J, et al. New transtracheal bronchoalveolar lavage technique for the diagnosis of respiratory disease in sheep. Vet Rec 2005;157(11):309–13.
24. Larsen LE, Tjornehoj K, Viuff B, et al. Diagnosis of enzootic pneumonia in Danish cattle: reverse transcription-polymerase chain reaction assay for detection of bovine respiratory syncytial virus in naturally and experimentally infected cattle. J Vet Diagn Invest 1999;11(5):416–22.
25. Kimman TG, Terpstra GK, Daha MR, et al. Pathogenesis of naturally acquired bovine respiratory syncytial virus infection in calves: evidence for the involvement of complement and mast cell mediators. Am J Vet Res 1989;50(5):694–700.

26. Webster JD, Miller MA, DuSold D, et al. Effects of prolonged formalin fixation on the immunohistochemical detection of infectious agents in formalin-fixed, paraffin-embedded tissues. Vet Pathol 2010;47(3):529–35.

27. Benavides J, Garcia-Pariente C, Gelmetti D, et al. Effects of fixative type and fixation time on the detection of maedi visna virus by PCR and immunohistochemistry in paraffin-embedded ovine lung samples. J Virol Methods 2006;137(2):317–24.

28. Ramos-Vara JA. Technical aspects of immunohistochemistry. Vet Pathol 2005; 42(4):405–26.

29. Decaro N, Buonavoglia C. Canine parvovirus: a review of epidemiological and diagnostic aspects, with emphasis on type 2c. Vet Microbiol 2012;155(1): 1–12.

30. Willoughby K, Thomson K, Maley M, et al. Development of a real time reverse transcriptase polymerase chain reaction for the detection of bovine respiratory syncytial virus in clinical samples and its comparison with immunohistochemistry and immunofluorescence antibody testing. Vet Microbiol 2008;126(1–3): 264–70.

31. Timsit E, Le Drean E, Maingourd C, et al. Detection by real-time RT-PCR of a bovine respiratory syncytial virus vaccine in calves vaccinated intranasally. Vet Rec 2009;165(8):230–3.

32. Eysker M. The sensitivity of the Baermann method for the diagnosis of primary Dictyocaulus viviparus infections in calves. Vet Parasitol 1997;69(1–2):89–93.

33. Wieringa L, van Dreumel T, Godkin A, et al. Unusual clinical signs in cattle associated with viral infection. Newsletter of the Animal Health Laboratory. University of Guelph; 2005.

34. Salman MD, Frank GR, MacVean DW, et al. Validation of disease diagnoses reported to the National Animal Health Monitoring System from a large Colorado beef feedlot. J Am Vet Med Assoc 1988;192(8):1069–73.

35. Buhman MJ, Perino LJ, Galyean ML, et al. Association between changes in eating and drinking behaviors and respiratory tract disease in newly arrived calves at a feedlot. Am J Vet Res 2000;61(10):1163–8.

36. Wittum TE, Woollen NE, Perino LJ, et al. Relationships among treatment for respiratory tract disease, pulmonary lesions evident at slaughter, and rate of weight gain in feedlot cattle. J Am Vet Med Assoc 1996;209(4):814–8.

37. White BJ, Renter DG. Bayesian estimation of the performance of using clinical observations and harvest lung lesions for diagnosing bovine respiratory disease in post-weaned beef calves. J Vet Diagn Invest 2009;21(4):446–53.

38. Gardner BA, Dolezal HG, Bryant LK, et al. Health of finishing steers: effects on performance, carcass traits, and meat tenderness. J Anim Sci 1999;77(12): 3168–75.

39. Thompson PN, Stone A, Schultheiss WA. Use of treatment records and lung lesion scoring to estimate the effect of respiratory disease on growth during early and late finishing periods in South African feedlot cattle. J Anim Sci 2006;84(2): 488–98.

40. Reinhold P, Rabeling B, Gunther H, et al. Comparative evaluation of ultrasonography and lung function testing with the clinical signs and pathology of calves inoculated experimentally with Pasteurella multocida. Vet Rec 2002;150(4): 109–14.

41. Ollivett TL, Burton AJ, Bicalho RC, et al. Use of rapid thoracic ultrasonography for detection of subclinical and clinical pneumonia in dairy calves. Proceedings of the American association of bovine practitioners 44th annual meeting. St Louis (MO); 2011. p. 148.

42. Hanzlicek GA, White BJ, Mosier D, et al. Serial evaluation of physiologic, pathological, and behavioral changes related to disease progression of experimentally induced Mannheimia haemolytica pneumonia in postweaned calves. Am J Vet Res 2010;71(3):359–69.

43. Thomson RG, Chander S, Savan M, et al. Investigation of factors of probable significance in the pathogenesis of pneumonic pasteurellosis in cattle. Can J Comp Med 1975;39(2):194–207.

44. Coghe J, Uystepruyst CH, Bureau F, et al. Validation and prognostic value of plasma lactate measurement in bovine respiratory disease. Vet J 2000;160(2): 139–46.

45. Godson DL, Campos M, Attah-Poku SK, et al. Serum haptoglobin as an indicator of the acute phase response in bovine respiratory disease. Vet Immunol Immunopathol 1996;51(3–4):277–92.

46. Carter JN, Meredith GL, Montelongo M, et al. Relationship of vitamin E supplementation and antimicrobial treatment with acute-phase protein responses in cattle affected by naturally acquired respiratory tract disease. Am J Vet Res 2002;63(8):1111–7.

47. Humblet MF, Coghe J, Lekeux P, et al. Acute phase proteins assessment for an early selection of treatments in growing calves suffering from bronchopneumonia under field conditions. Res Vet Sci 2004;77(1):41–7.

48. Ganheim C, Hulten C, Carlsson U, et al. The acute phase response in calves experimentally infected with bovine viral diarrhoea virus and/or Mannheimia haemolytica. J Vet Med B Infect Dis Vet Public Health 2003;50(4):183–90.

49. Heegaard PM, Godson DL, Toussaint MJ, et al. The acute phase response of haptoglobin and serum amyloid A (SAA) in cattle undergoing experimental infection with bovine respiratory syncytial virus. Vet Immunol Immunopathol 2000; 77(1–2):151–9.

50. Knobloch H, Schroedl W, Turner C, et al. Electronic nose responses and acute phase proteins correlate in blood using a bovine model of respiratory infection. Sens Actuators B Chem 2010;144(1):81–7.

51. Svensson C, Liberg P, Hultgren J. Evaluating the efficacy of serum haptoglobin concentration as an indicator of respiratory-tract disease in dairy calves. Vet J 2007;174(2):288–94.

52. Angen O, Thomsen J, Larsen LE, et al. Respiratory disease in calves: microbiological investigations on trans-tracheally aspirated bronchoalveolar fluid and acute phase protein response. Vet Microbiol 2009;137(1–2):165–71.

53. Orro T, Pohjanvirta T, Rikula U, et al. Acute phase protein changes in calves during an outbreak of respiratory disease caused by bovine respiratory syncytial virus. Comp Immunol Microbiol Infect Dis 2011;34(1):23–9.

Diagnostics of Dairy and Beef Cattle Diarrhea

Patricia Carey Blanchard, DVM, PhD

KEYWORDS

- Calf diarrhea • *Cryptosporidium* • Coronavirus • Rotavirus • *E coli* • *Salmonella*

KEY POINTS

- Calf diarrhea is a multifactorial disease related to a combination of host and pathogen factors.
- The most common pathogens found in diarrheic calves are *Cryptosporidium*, rotavirus, coronavirus, *Salmonella*, attaching and effacing *Escherichia coli* (enterohemorrhagic *Escherichia coli* [EHEC], enteropathogenic *Escherichia coli* [EPEC], Shiga toxin–producing *Escherichia coli* [STEC]), and F5 (K99) *E coli*.
- Increased mortality and morbidity are often due to the presence of more than one pathogen.
- Identifying subsets of affected animals via farm interviews and record review may lead to key factors in which intervention could prevent future cases.

INTRODUCTION

The clinical history can be an important tool in the diagnosis, prevention, and treatment of causes of calf diarrhea. The age of onset of diarrhea is an important factor in ruling in or out some agents. F5 (K99) *E coli* typically causes diarrhea in calves less than 6-days old, whereas *Cryptosporidium* will not be detectable in the feces before 3-days old and coccidia not before 15 to 21 days due to their prepatent periods. The presence of blood in the feces of calves less than 30-days old is most commonly associated with *Salmonella*, coronavirus, attaching and effacing *E coli*, and, rarely, *Cryptosporidium* and *Clostridium*.

Identifying subsets of affected animals via farm interviews and record review may lead to key factors in which intervention could prevent future cases. For instance, in a dairy situation, if affected calves are disproportionately born in the evening, weekends, or holidays, this might indicate inadequate training of some personnel responsible for ensuring calves receive colostrum and are moved to a clean, dry area (calf

The author has nothing to disclose.
University of California Animal Health and Food Safety Laboratory, School of Veterinary Medicine, University of California-Davis, 18830 Road 112, Tulare, CA 93274, USA
E-mail address: pcblanchard@ucdavis.edu

Vet Clin Food Anim 28 (2012) 443–464

hutch, calf pen or clean cow-calf area). When most affected calves are the offspring of primiparous heifers and the dams' colostrum is fed to calves, this might indicate dry cow vaccines (rotavirus, coronavirus, and K99 *E coli*) that are used in multiparous cows have not been given to first-calving heifers. First-calf heifers may also have lower quality and quantity of colostrum. In beef cow-calf operations, use of pens for calving and nursing cows may lead to build up of pathogens shed by cows and their calves over the duration of the calving season, thereby exposing newborn calves to higher pathogen loads and increasing the likelihood of their developing diarrhea. The calving pen or calf housing may be a source of pathogens that persist from year to year in moist cool areas.

The source of milk may be a factor if hospital milk with antibiotics or unpasteurized milk with pathogens (ie, *Salmonella*) is fed to calves. The pasteurizer might be over-heating and degrading the milk quality or not reaching sufficient time and temperature to kill pathogens. Diarrhea outbreaks following the purchase of a new lot, source, or type of calf milk replacer might indicate product quality problems.

Sentinel bull calves may be used when calf diarrhea results in high morbidity but low mortality and when the owner is unwilling to sacrifice a potential replacement heifer calf. Sentinel calves should have necropsies performed within 1 to 2 days after onset of diarrhea at the age when other calves on the premise are also affected. To improve detection of pathogens, these calves should not be treated with any therapeutics besides electrolytes and supportive therapy. Transport and comingling of calves from multiple premises may result in exposure to pathogens to which some calves may not have colostral immunity. Purchase of calves less than 30-days old can bring pathogens on to a farm and expose a naïve population of cows and calves.

Response to antibiotic treatment would support the presence of a bacterial compo-nent. Bacterial overgrowth secondary to undigested feed in the lower intestine may show some response to antibiotics, even though the primary cause is villus atrophy from a viral or *Cryptosporidium* infection. An antibiotic treatment failure does not rule out bacterial causes because the organism may be resistant or the antibiotic may not attain adequate distribution and therapeutic levels to kill bacteria in the intes-tinal lumen. Use of antibiotics on nonbacterial diarrheas may worsen the diarrhea by suppressing the normal flora, which could allow yeast, *Salmonella*, and attaching and effacing *E coli* to overgrow.

FIELD NECROPSY FOR CALF DIARRHEA

Calves should be assessed for presence of dehydration because dehydrated calves may no longer have evidence of the diarrhea. Other causes of dehydration, such as prolonged lack of fluid intake or renal disease, can be ruled out by the history and gross and histologic evaluation of kidneys. During the necropsy, note the presence or absence of fat stores around the kidney and size of the thymus. These observations give an indication of the length of time the animal has been ill. Decreased fat stores are more common in 10- to 21-day old calves, particularly in cold, wet weather.

Examine the oral cavity and esophagus for evidence of erosion, proliferation (bovine papular stomatitis virus), and bruises. Examine the contents of the forestomachs. Unusual color (eg, pink, green) or texture (gelatinous) of contents may indicate the use of oral medications. White plaques progressing to curd like attachments on the rumen, reticulum, or omasum mucosa are commonly seen with yeast infections. Small, often red, raised foci may be present in the rumen mucosa and this is a nonspe-cific vesicular and suppurative change. Determine if there is fermenting milk or curd in the rumen because this can cause mucosal irritation. Assess the position, size, color, thickness, and texture of the abomasum. Reddening and edema often indicate inflammation, black linear ulcers or round deep ulcers should be noted and collected for histopathology (see later discussion).

Examination of the small intestine should include spot checks of areas with different color, thickness, and contents. Place 1 cm, partially opened sections of four different areas of the small intestine into formalin. Include the following areas: one duodenum, one midjejunum, one between midjejunum and distal ileum, and, the last, and most important, the ileum at the ileocecal ligament (**Fig. 1**). Collect a second section of ileum to be submitted unfixed. Examine the cecum, which may have a full thickness infarct on the antimesenteric border or a circumferential infarct. These lesions are of undetermined cause. The cecum may have milder lesions similar to the spiral colon. Spiral colon sections should be submitted both fresh and fixed with two loops (2 cm) attached to each other to identify the tissue as spiral colon (see later discussion). The descending colon should also be examined and, if abnormal, a section submitted for histopathology. Collect 2 to 5 mL of feces in a tube or bag for fecal tests because the contents remaining in the spiral colon alone may be insufficient for all the testing needed. See **Table 1** for suggested samples to submit from field necropsies.

TECHNIQUES FOR DIAGNOSIS OF PATHOGENS

There is no one test that will detect a pathogen with 100% accuracy. **Table 2** lists a summary of diarrhea pathogens, specimen, and types of tests available. Each test method has limitations; the laboratory to which the veterinarian submits samples should be able to provide this information. Case-control studies and fecal surveys have detected all enteric pathogens associated with calf diarrhea in calves that do not have diarrhea. Both host and pathogen factors influence the severity and likelihood a calf will develop diarrhea. The major host factors include the general health, nutrition, immunity to specific pathogens, and age of exposure. The major pathogen factors include the number of infectious particles, number of concurrent diseases, and virulence of the agent. For this reason, it is incumbent on the clinician to interpret the detection of pathogens in the context of the signs and clinical history. Necropsy and histopathology of good quality tissues can aid in determining the role of an agent in causing diarrhea by the detection of lesions in the tissues associated with that agent.

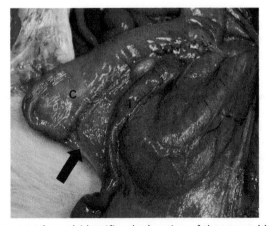

Fig. 1. Ileocecal ligament (*arrow*) identifies the location of the cecum (c) and ileum (i).

Table 1
Suggested tissues to collect and submit from field necropsies

Tissue	Size	Container	Use
Lung Liver	8 × 6 × 6 cm	Bag (separate)	Culture (for sepsis) Toxicology
Ileum (at ileocecal ligament)	2 cm long	Bag (separate)	Culture FA
Spiral colon (2 attached loops)	2 cm long	Bag (separate)	Culture FA
Feces	2–5 mL	Bag (separate)	Culture EM agELISA Lateral flow Etc
Ileum (at ileocecal ligament) Midjejunum and distal jejunum Duodenum (1each)	1 cm (part open)	10% formalin	Histopathology
Spiral colon (2 attached loops)	1 cm long (part open)	10% formalin	Histopathology
Lung Heart Liver kidney Thymus Spleen	1 × 1 × 1 cm	10% formalin	Histopathology
Lesion (fresh and fixed)	—	Fresh and 10% formalin	Testing as appropriate

Molecular diagnostics, most often polymerase chain reaction (PCR)-based tests, are becoming more common in diagnostic laboratories and present their own challenges in interpretation. PCR methods are usually more sensitive ($\sim 10^3$ organisms/mL) than antigen-detection methods (10^4–10^7 organisms/mL), such as ELISA, fluorescent antibody (FA), agglutination, and chromatography (lateral flow, dipstick); and more sensitive than direct visualization (10^6–10^7 organisms/mL), such as electron microscopy (EM), fecal flotation, or stained fecal smears.[1,2] However, PCR methods may miss viruses or bacteria that have mutated or drifted from the sequence specific to the primers in use.[1] PCR methods may detect lower levels of pathogens that may not be causing disease due to age resistance (F5 [K99] *E coli*) or may detect the pathogen after the signs of illness have resolved.[2] PCR methods detect pathogens even in the presence of antibody-antigen complexes. However, if the agent is bound to antibody, it is less likely to be causing disease, so detection by PCR may overestimate its significance. PCR methods may fail to detect an agent due to inhibitory substances in the sample, which is more likely to occur in fecal samples than in lung or nasal swabs. Newer methods to extract nucleic acid have overcome many of the problems posed by testing of feces for organisms such as *Salmonella*, making PCR as sensitive as culture. However, the sensitivity of each method may vary with the species of *Salmonella* found in the sample.[1,3] Dead or stressed bacteria can be detected by PCR in samples in which they might not grow in cultures.[3] Sample quality, quantity, appropriate type, storage, and transport are all important issues to be aware of when submitting samples for PCR to ensure the pathogen of interest is not denatured or

Table 2
Detection methods and specimen type for the diagnosis of calf diarrhea agents

Pathogen	Specimen	Test Methods
Clostridium perfringens Type C	Small intestine contents (frozen)	Culture and genotyping, toxin: agELISA, PCR
Clostridium difficile	Feces (if alive)	HP (tissue)
	Intestine lesion (fixed)	Culture and toxin testing
	Colon contents or feces (fresh or frozen)	HP (tissue)
	Colon and ileum (fixed)	
E coli, K99 (F5)	Feces and/or ileum content	agELISA
	Ileum (fixed)	Culture
		IC, LA, SA, PCR
		HP
E coli, attaching and effacing	Ileum and colon (fresh and fixed)	HP and culture (typing, PCR eae gene and/or toxin detection)
Salmonella spp	Feces	Culture, IC, PCR
	Intestine	
	Tissues	
Coronavirus	Colon and ileum (fresh-FA)	FA, HP
	Feces	agELISA, EM, IC, PCR
Rotavirus	Feces, small intestine (fresh- FA)	agELISA, EM, FA, IC, LA, PCR
Cryptosporidium spp	Feces	AF, agELISA, FA, Flotation, IC, PCR
Coccidia	Feces	Flotation, McMaster's
	Colon	HP, scraping- direct (unfixed)
Nematodes	Feces	Flotation, McMaster's
	Abomasum, intestine	Gross examination
Septicemia	Lung and/or liver (fresh)	Culture
Copper deficiency	Liver	ICP-AES or AA
	Serum	

Abbreviations: AA, atomic absorption; AF, acid-fast stain on direct smear; agELISA, antigen ELIZA; EM, electron microscopy; FA, fluorescent antibody test; HP, histopathology; IC, immune-chromatography assay (lateral-flow agELISA); ICP, inductively coupled plasma atomic emission spectroscopy; LA, latex agglutination; PCR, polymerase chain reaction with nucleic acid probe; SA, slide agglutination.

destroyed. PCR methods will increase the detection of low levels of organisms that arise from cross-contamination from one calf to another when fecal samples are collected using the same instruments to open the intestinal tract or while wearing the same pair of examination gloves to collect feces from multiple animals. If the goal is simply to determine the presence of the agent in a group of animals, cross-contamination is less of a concern on the same premise than if the goal is to determine the prevalence of agents in clinically affected animals to prioritize prevention strategies. Cleaning instruments well between premises is vital to ensure agents are not detected on a premise where they do not exist due to use of contaminated instruments from another premise.

EM has been used for virus detection in feces for decades. This technique requires approximately 10^6 to 10^7 particles/g or ml of feces for detection, although this level can be reduced by the use of immunoelectron microscopy.[4] Particle integrity, the likelihood to become damaged in processing or during storage so as to make it unidentifiable, or the presence of cell material that can look like the virus particle, can cause false negative or false positive results particularly for coronaviruses.[1,4] EM, like virus isolation, has the unique ability to detect novel viruses or viruses for which there is no diagnostic assay. The drawback is that EM does not always allow the determination of the type of virus, particularly when small round viruses are detected. These viruses may have no specific visual characteristic that differentiate them from among several types of viruses in the same size range.

Antigen-detection assays (ELISA, agglutination, immune-chromatography, immunohistochemistry [IHC], and FA) are based on detection of conserved antigens (often proteins) found among a heterologous agent population. Their advantage is they allow detection of a wide array of similar agents. For instance, group A rotavirus ELISA assays designed for human medicine will detect group A rotavirus in many species including calves.[2] A disadvantage is that the host or colostrum antibody binding to the antigen will inhibit detection. However, calves with antibody may not develop illness because their immune response is preventing or resolving the infection.

Culture methods on feces using enrichment broth for *Salmonella* may detect isolates missed by PCR and vice versa.[1,3] The precollection use of antibiotics and overgrowth of normal flora or altered flora, particularly in samples that are not freshly collected, may lead to failure to detect the pathogen by culture. Virus isolation is particularly difficult on feces due to the presence of bacteria and other agents that may be toxic to cell cultures.

INFECTIOUS CAUSES OF DIARRHEA IN CALVES LESS THAN 3-MONTHS OLD

The most common causes of diarrhea reported in calves less than 30-days old are rotavirus and *Cryptosporidium*.[5,6] **Table 3** shows the agents in the frequency they

Table 3
CAHFS-Tulare 4-year (2008–2011) summary of enteric pathogens, production type, and age (mean and range) from 2311 necropsied calves less than 35-days old with diarrhea

Pathogen	Positive (%)	Mean Age (Days)	Age Range (Days)
Cryptosporidium sp	37.2	13.0	3–33
Coronavirus	30.5	10.4	1–30
Rotavirus	26.6	10.5	1–32
Salmonella spp:	15.7	—	—
Salmonella group D1 (*S dublin*)	5.8	17.1	2–30
Salmonella group C2 (*S newport*)	4.2	8.7	1–30
Salmonella group B (*S typhimurium*)	2.7	8.1	1–30
Salmonella group E	2.3	12.6	2–21
Salmonella C1 and not grouped	0.7	—	—
Attaching and effacing *E coli*	10.5	12.0	1–31
K99 *E coli*	4.5	2.3	1–7
Bovine viral diarrhea virus	1.3	16.1	2–30
Production type	%	—	—
Calf ranch	62	—	—
Dairy	33	—	—
Beef	2	—	—
Not reported/Other	3	—	—

were detected, mean age, age range, and production type from calves less than 35-days old submitted over a 4-year period (January 2008–January 2012) to the California Animal Health and Food Safety Laboratory (CAHFS) in Tulare. Only cases in which whole calves or tissues from calves including ileum and colon were submitted were included. These data show coronavirus as the second most common pathogen, unlike several other studies based on testing of feces from live animals. This may reflect a higher mortality due to coronavirus or, possibly, a more sensitive detection method using FA on colon tissue compared with methods used on feces only (ELISA, EM). Like other studies, most calves had more than one pathogen detected. More than 95% of these animals originated from calf ranches or dairies. Fecal only submissions were excluded because coronavirus and attaching and effacing E coli could not be evaluated in those animals.

After 30-days of age, *Salmonella dublin*, coccidia, and occasionally rumen acidosis are the more common causes of diarrhea. Bovine viral diarrhea virus (BVDv) and abomasal parasitism in pasture calves occurs most often after 3-months of age.

CLOSTRIDIUM PERFRINGENS TYPE C AND CLOSTRIDIUM DIFFICILE

Clostridium perfringens type C is a rare cause of enteritis or diarrhea in calves less than 10-days old. The gross pathologic lesions in the small intestine are hemorrhagic and necrotizing. If diarrhea is present, there will be blood or a red color to the feces. The major differentials when performing a necropsy of a calf that has died of *C perfringens* type C is a mesenteric root torsion, segmental intestinal volvulus, intestinal entrapment, or a severe *Salmonella* infection. Confirmatory diagnosis of this infection requires the detection of beta and alpha toxin in intestinal contents. Intestine contents from dead animals or feces from live animal should be frozen as soon as possible to prevent the breakdown of the toxin. In some cases, only beta toxin will be detected and these should also be considered strong evidence of *C perfringens* type C presence. Isolation of *C perfringens* alone is not diagnostic unless genotyping reveals the organisms are type C. Normal flora includes *C perfringens* type A, which has also been reported to cause gastroenteritis in calves. Typical gross and histologic lesions of small intestine necrosis, hemorrhage, suppurative inflammation, and large numbers of large gram-positive rods provides a strong presumptive diagnosis of *C perfringens* type C.

Clostridium difficile toxins have been shown experimentally and naturally to be associated with small intestinal villus tip degeneration and superficial colon erosion with fibrin and neutrophil and eosinophil exudate. Experimentally purified toxin B caused more severe small intestine and colon ulceration. Both the toxin and organism (by culture) have been found in diarrhea and nondiarrhea calves.[7]

E COLI, ATTACHING AND EFFACING

Moxley and Smith[8] wrote an excellent review of the literature of experimental and natural infection and epidemiologic studies related to finding attaching and effacing *E coli* (AEEC; with intimin [eae] genes) with or without Shiga toxin (also known as verotoxin), Stx1 or Stx2 genes, and Shiga toxin–producing *Escherichia coli* (STEC) without the eae genes. Using the human literature definitions, *E coli* with both Shiga toxin and eae genes are considered enterohemorrhagic *Escherichia coli* (EHEC) and include O157:H7, which can be found in cattle as carriers and has been shown to attach and cause diarrhea in some studies.[8] *E coli* with the eae genes but no Shiga toxin genes are referred to as enteropathogenic *Escherichia coli* (EPEC). All three groups (EHEC, EPEC, and STEC) have been found in diarrhea calves with natural infections and have been used successfully to reproduce enteritis and/or colitis in some, but not all, inoculated calves. Several studies demonstrated that calves less than 24-hours old without colostral antibodies are more likely to develop diarrhea and intestinal lesions when inoculated with the organisms than are older calves or calves that have received colostrum.[8] Epidemiologic studies that are stratified by age also show as much as 10 to 12 times higher recovery of AEEC or STEC-type organisms in calves less than 30-days old with diarrhea compared with controls without diarrhea.[8] In calves over 30-days old or in reports in which calves of all ages were clustered, as well as in adult animals, there is either no difference or only an approximately twofold difference in fecal detection rates between diarrhea and nondiarrhea animals.[8,9] Based on histologic confirmation, AEEC organisms most often cause diarrhea in calves between 2- to 21-days old with a mean age of 10 to 12 days.[8,10–12] Occasional cases have been reported in calves up to 4-months old and adults.[8,10–12] Following experimental inoculation, onset of diarrhea ranged from 1 to 4 days and lasted for 1 to 7 days.[8] In some studies, calves had onset of a mild fever (up to 40°C) between 36 hours and 4 days postinoculation that lasted 1 to 3 days. However, experimentally, the onset and severity of clinical signs are influenced by specific type of E coli, dosage, age at exposure, and colostral immunity. The literature suggests the same is true of natural infections.

The confirmatory diagnosis of AEEC is by microscopic examination of the small intestine and colon. Janke and colleagues[10,12] observed attachment in the colon In 88.4% of cases, which included 31.7% of cases with both small intestine (ileum) and colon attachment, only 11.7% of cases had attachment in the small intestine alone. AEEC cause a distinct histologic appearance at the attachment sites where clusters of short gram-negative rods attach and form a scalloped appearance to the epithelial cells (**Fig. 2**).[8,10,12] These cells undergo damage to their microvillus surface, round up, degenerate, and slough from the lamina propria. When the small intestine is affected, villus atrophy results from loss of affected cells. Inflammation may be mild but varies with duration of the lesion.[8] On gross necropsy, the colon mucosa may be normal or have longitudinal reddening, roughening, and petechial hemorrhages (**Fig. 3**).[8] Blood flecks, attached clots, or frank hemorrhage, mucus, and fibrin are also seen in some calves.[8] Occasional cases may develop a pseudomembrane in the small intestine. The gross findings are not specific to AEEC and may be seen with coronavirus and Salmonella in calves less than 30-days old. Feces can vary in color and consistency. Some calves will have watery yellow feces, whereas others

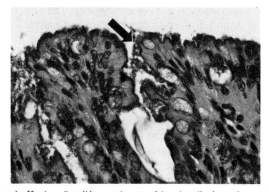

Fig. 2. Attaching and effacing E coli bacteria attaching in piled up clumps (arrow) on surface epithelium resulting in scalloped irregular surface. H and E slide 1000×.

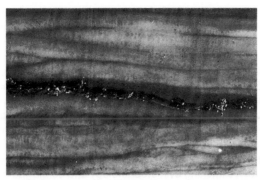

Fig. 3. Attaching and effacing *E coli* resulting in hemorrhage and roughening of mucosa with fibrin in lumen of spiral colon. The same lesion could be seen with coronavirus or *Salmonella*.

may have blood in the feces, which is most common with EHEC strains.[8,10,12] In some calves, the feces may appear near normal, probably due to dehydration (Pat Blanchard, unpublished observation). The cecum and descending colon or rectum may have lesions when the spiral colon does not.[8]

Optimal diagnostic detection is gained by histopathology of the ileum near the ileo-cecal junction and at least two loops of spiral colon and, when gross lesions are noted, sections of cecum and descending colon or rectum. Samples submitted for histopathology should have minimal handling to prevent removal of the affected surface epithelium. Formalin-fixed sections should be partially opened to allow entry of formalin into the lumen. Do not tie off sections placed in formalin because this slows formalin fixation of the mucosa unless the ligated tissue has been filled with formalin.

AEEC has also been reported as the sole pathogen detected in 17% to 35% of cases in three reports.[10–12] These reports found 51% to 64% of isolates produced verotoxin (Shiga toxin) though higher percent of toxin-producing strains associated with diarrhea have been reported by others.[8] In one review, 27% of AEEC-affected calves were also septicemic.[11] Occasionally, veterinarians request an antimicrobial sensitivity of the attaching organism. To confirm an *E coli* isolated from the intestine is an attaching and effacing strain, PCR screening for the presence of the eae or toxin genes (Stx1, Stx2) is needed. A small in-house study at the authors' laboratory, found 85% of calves with moderate to large number of attaching organisms in the colon had the eae gene in 9 to 10 of 10 isolates selected from the 4+ growth zone of a colon swab plated on MacConkey agar; whereas only two of four calves had the eae gene in 1 to 2 of 10 isolates and the other two had no isolates with the eae gene when rare to small number of organisms were seen attaching (Pat Blanchard, unpublished observation). These findings indicate that random selection of an *E coli* from the 4+ growth zone of a colon mucosal swab is likely to yield an attaching and effacing strain when there are moderate to large number of organisms seen attaching histologically.

ENTEROTOXIGENIC *E COLI* (F5 [K99])

Enterotoxigenic *E coli* bacteria possess the fimbrial antigen F5 often referred to as K99. The fimbria allows the bacteria to attach to the villus epithelial cells of the small intestine and secrete a toxin. After attaching, the heat stable toxin (STa) acts on the epithelial cells to result in marked fluid efflux into the small intestine lumen.[13] The attachment factors are most commonly expressed on immature villus epithelial cells. Therefore, normal postnatal maturation limits the disease potential of this organism to calves usually less than 6-days old.[13,14] There may be periods of increased suscepti-bility after 5-days old if calves experience villus atrophy from other causes (viruses and *Cryptosporidium*) resulting in immature cells migrating from the crypts to cover the villus tips.[13] In one study testing only feces from calves with diarrhea, 17 of 26 animals with F5 *E coli* isolated had concurrent infection with *Cryptosporidium*, rotavirus, and/or coronavirus.[15] F5 *E coli* were found in all ages up to 30 days, but the authors did not indicate if the animals with F5 *E coli* isolated after 5-days old were the same ones with concurrent other pathogens. Unfortunately, most published prevalence studies are based on testing feces from diarrhea and nondiarrhea calves; therefore, there is no histopathology to show the organism is attaching. In **Table 3**, the mean age of 2.5 days and age range of 1 to 7 days for K99 (F5) *E coli* is based on necropsies in which the organism was seen attaching by histopathology and confirmed by latex agglutina-tion on feces or isolates.

The fluid loss into the intestine (**Fig. 4**) with this disease may be so severe that calves die of dehydration and electrolyte imbalance before diarrhea is detected. In some cases, the diarrhea may go unnoticed due to the very thin watery nature being mistaken for urine or seeping rapidly into the bedding. The feeding of colostrum from cows vaccinated with F5 (K99)–specific antigen is effective in preventing the disease. Once an outbreak occurs, if dry cow vaccines are not in use, oral products containing F5 (K99) specific antibodies can also be used to prevent attachment until colostral antibodies are available from cows vaccinated 10 days or more prepartum.

The presence of F5 (K99) *E coli* can be detected by isolation and typing, PCR, or antigen-detection methods (ELISA, immunochromatography, slide, or latex agglutina-tion). Test methods with lower sensitivity are more likely to detect the organism when it is causing diarrhea because higher numbers will be present when it attaches to the epithelium. More sensitive methods, such as PCR and even culture, will find the organism in calves in which it may not be causing disease, but this provides informa-tion about the presence of the bacteria on the premise.

Other enterotoxigenic *E coli*, F41 and 987P, are occasionally reported in calves with diarrhea and when present will have a similar histologic lesion to F5 (K99) *E coli* but F5 (K99)–detection methods would be negative for these organisms. However, methods that detect presence of heat-stable toxin (STa) would identify the possible presence of these uncommon organisms. Histopathology of freshly collected and formalin-fixed sections of ileum will have typical attachment of medium-size gram-negative bacterial

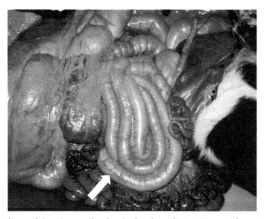

Fig. 4. F5 (K99) *E coli* resulting in marked spiral colon distention with watery yellow content (*arrow*).

rods inserting into the brush border of the villus epithelial cells with morphologically normal epithelial cells. Often there is very little inflammation.

SALMONELLA SP

Enteric *Salmonella* infections can result in the full gamut of gross lesions ranging from watery yellow feces to hemorrhage, necrosis, fibrin casts, and pseudomembrane (**Fig. 5**) or lesions similar to those described earlier for attaching and effacing *E coli*. Abomasal reddening, roughening, and exudates may also be present, although these are nonspecific changes. Enlarged mesenteric lymph nodes are often seen (see **Fig. 5**). The most common causes of enteric *Salmonella* infections in calves less than 21-days old are *Salmonella typhimurium* (serogroup B) and *Salmonella newport* (serogroup C2)[16] (Pat Blanchard unpublished observation). However, disease with other serotypes have been described (**Table 3**). Both these agents are also common causes of diarrhea in cows in the first 5 days after parturition. *Salmonella* serogroups C1 and E may be found in calves the first few days of life and can be transient colonizers in calves without diarrhea.[17] These serogroups (C1 and E) and others (C3, F, G, K) less often associated with diarrhea may also be found on dairies in the environment, feed, water sources (eg, creeks, standing water, lagoons, troughs), and feces of nondiarrheic animals, rodents, and wildlife.[18] Pathogenic types like *S typhimurium*, *S newport*, and *S dublin* are also found at a lower rate.[17,18] Bacteremia and septicemia with *Salmonella* serogroups other than group D1 are usually late-onset events and probably result from invasion of the organism through necrotic areas of intestinal mucosa.

S dublin (serogroup D1), a cattle-adapted serotype, causes septicemia often as the primary and, sometimes, only disease condition. However, more often, some degree of enteritis is present histologically even in the absence of diarrhea. In some cases, the primary disease is enteric with diarrhea similar to *S newport* and *S typhimurium*. *S dublin* can cause diarrhea in calves as young as 5-days old but, more commonly, it occurs in calves from 1- to 4-months old.[19] A typical history is that calves show respiratory signs, diarrhea, illthrift, and have a poor response to antibiotics used for

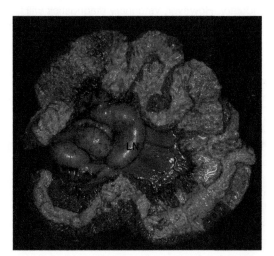

Fig. 5. *Salmonella newport* or *S typhimurium* infection related pseudomembrane on mucosa of small intestine and enlarged mesenteric lymph nodes (LN).

common causes of bronchopneumonia. Outbreaks can occur with high morbidity and mortality. Lesions of *S dublin* septicemia commonly include splenomegaly; hepatomegaly with a bronze coloration to the liver, lungs that fail to collapse on opening the chest cavity with hundreds of petechial hemorrhages; or plum-colored, wet and heavy (meaty texture) lungs involving caudal lobes; one or more cranial lobes; or all lobes (**Fig. 6**). On occasion, lesions will be limited to the cranial lung but, histologically, these lesions, like the wet, heavy lung, are due to variable amounts of fibrin, some forming hyaline membranes, and interstitial pneumonia with neutrophils and histiocytes. A single plug (coagulum of fibrin and bile) may be found in the gall bladder of some calves (**Fig. 7**) and is pathognomonic for *Salmonella* septicemia. Some calves may be icteric or have petechial hemorrhages in the kidney and gastrointestinal serosa. A few calves will have meningitis or polyarthritis. A rare dry gangrene condition associated with *S dublin* may be seen in winter months. Dry gangrene develops in the tips of the ears, tail, and both rear legs. In the legs, a sharp line of demarcation may form across the midmetatarsus or the gangrene may be limited to the phalanges. The foot may fall off. Lesions are similar to those seen with ergot but are linked to vascular thrombosis due to *S dublin*. The organism can usually be isolated from the feces of some affected calves though classic septicemia lesions are not present. *S dublin* can be carried by healthy cows and shed sporadically in milk and feces.[20] It is possible that young calves harbor the organism in their intestine or mesenteric lymph nodes until colostral antibodies wane, allowing it to spread.

Detection of *Salmonella* sp may be done by culture of mesenteric lymph nodes, intestinal lesions or contents, feces, and affected parenchymal organs. *Salmonella* cultures often involve one or more enrichment steps followed by PCR, lateral-flow chromatography, or isolation on selective media. Laboratories performing nonisolation methods, such as PCR, may follow positive results with isolation by request— or this may be done routinely. False negative PCR or isolation may occur due to suppression of growth in enrichment broth by normal intestinal flora or use of antibiotics in the animal so the organism may be present in numbers too few to detect. PCR methods on intestine may be impacted by release of enzymes from other bacteria that damage the nucleic acid of *Salmonella* sp making them undetectable.[1] Rapid, accurate detection methods continue to be developed and improved, primarily driven by the food industry. However, veterinary diagnostics will benefit from spinoff use of some of this technology to provide cost-effective, sensitive, and rapid detection of *Salmonella*.

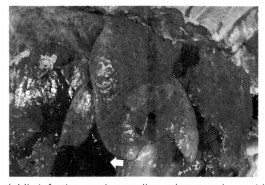

Fig. 6. *Salmonella dublin* infection causing swollen, edematous lung with petechial hemorrhages and localized areas of slightly firm (meaty) bronchointerstitial pneumonia (*arrow*).

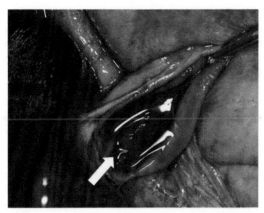

Fig. 7. *Salmonella dublin* infection a bile plug (fibrin) (*arrow*) in the edematous gall bladder.

In the face of a *Salmonella* outbreak in calves, all potential sources of spread should be considered and evaluated for possible sources of exposure. These include fomites on clothes, footwear, equipment, or feeding supplies (bottles, buckets, esophageal tubes—*Salmonella* can be found in saliva); as well as, water, colostrum, milk, conveyances (carts to remove dead calves and move newborn calves to hutches), wash water used in pens and under hutches, sprinklers, weigh scales, maternity pens, and sick cows.[20] Studies have shown increased fecal shedding in calves that did not receive antibiotic supplemented milk replacer,[17,19] on dairies where the maternity pen is used as a hospital pen,[19] when prophylactic antibiotics were given to newborn calves, and when the herd was not closed.[17] Reduced shedding and resistance to disease is seen with increasing age.[17,20]

CRYPTOSPORIDIUM

Cryptosporidium parvum, C bovis (formerly bovine B genotype),[21] *C ryanae* (formerly deer-like genotype),[22] and *C andersoni* have all been reported in calves.[23,24] Oocysts from *C bovis* and *C parvum* are indistinguishable based on size.[21] *C ryanae* oocysts are slightly smaller[22] and *C andersoni* are larger; the latter are primarily associated with subclinical disease from abomasal colonization in animals greater than 3-months old, usually adults. In a multistate study in the United States, *C parvum* was the primary species (~90% of *Cryptosporidium*) colonizing calves up to 4-weeks old and the only species found in calves less than 3-weeks old.[23] The peak prevalence of calves shedding *Cryptosporidium* was 66.7% at 2-weeks old when only *C parvum* was seen. *C parvum* only accounted for 1% of the *Cryptosporidium* found after weaning. *C bovis* and *C ryanae* were the most common types seen postweaning with peak postweaning shedding prevalence of 30% at 6-months old. The predominant species varies by region. *C bovis* was the most common type at all ages in Sweden where *C parvum* was only found in calves before weaning with 73% of *C parvum*–infected calves less than 2-weeks old.[24] Some reports in the literature show no statistical difference in shedding of *Cryptosporidium* between diarrhea and age-matched control calves; others report over 90% of calves shed the organism in the preweaning period.[6,25] Several surveys have found *Cryptosporidium* was the most common or second-most common pathogen in the feces of diarrhea calves. The authors' laboratory (see **Table 3**) and most surveys report over 35% of diarrheic calves less than 30-days old shedding this agent.[5,6,23,25–27] Like other enteric pathogens in calves,

Cryptosporidium has been associated with mixed infections; and a peak shedding prevalence at 7 to 14 days (53%–95%), both of which decline with increasing age.[6,26,27] Earlier surveillance studies did not determine the species of *Cryptosporidium* and often included calves older than 30-days old, which may explain the lack of correlation between shedding and diarrhea because some of the older calves may have been infected with *C bovis*.

Histopathology and experimental studies with *C parvum* demonstrate its attachment to the small intestine villus epithelial cells and resultant villus atrophy. In severe cases, the organism can be found in crypts in the colon accompanied by neutrophils. When the organism affects the colon it can lead to blood in the feces but this does not occur when found in the small intestine alone. The prepatent period for *C parvum* is 3 to 4 days, though first shedding is more often detected at 6- to 7-days old and can last 4 to 18 days. Most affected calves are 6- to 25-days old. *C bovis* has been identified in feces of calves as young as 7 days[24] and *C ryanae* at 11- to 12-days old.[21,24] These two species are most often associated with subclinical infection.[21,22,24]

Antigen detection methods, such as ELISA and chromatographic methods, probably detect all species of *Cryptosporidium* (A. Broes, personal communication, 2012) and FA have been shown to detect all species.[23] Visualization of oocysts via fecal flotation, direct examination, and acid-fast stains also will not distinguish *C parvum, C bovis*, and, to a lesser extent, *C ryanae* because they are all approximately the same size. PCR methods with 18S ribosomal RNA sequencing have been used to distinguish the four species of *Cryptosporidium* and subtypes of *C parvum* that are associated with human infection.[24] PCR methods can detect lower number of organisms (as low as 50–100/g but, more consistently, 250 oocysts/g)[24] than antigen detection (FA, ELISA, chromatography) and fecal flotation or acid-fast stained direct smears, which have detection limits ranging from 10^3 to 10^6 oocysts/g of feces. The lower limits are more often associated with concentration of oocysts before detection. Quantitation of the organism by direct examination, including acid-fast stains and flotation may be misleading because low numbers may reflect the stage of infection (early or late) instead of the severity. However, one study found calves shedding more than 2.2×10^5 oocysts/g of feces had a 6.1 times greater likelihood of having diarrhea than calves shedding lower numbers of organisms.[27]

Cryptosporidium are remarkably resistant to disinfectants, making them hard to kill and no effective therapeutics have been found. Five percent ammonia, 6% hydrogen peroxide, and 10% formalin are reported to kill the organism[20]; however, none of these are practical to use on farms. Increasing environmental temperatures from 4°C to 20°C[28,29] and the resultant higher temperatures found in fecal pats, which exceed 40°C, resulted in rapid inactivation of oocysts.[30] Likewise, reduced temperatures below −22°C also resulted in inactivation of oocysts.[28] Atwill and colleagues[25] found the organism could still be detected in scrapings from the walls and floor of wooden calf hutches after cleaning.

Szonyi and colleagues[31] determined calf age (less than 1-month old), housing calves in the cow barn, larger herd size (>200), use of hay bedding, and precipitation (100–150 mm) increased the risk of calves shedding *C parvum*: whereas increased slope (5%–10%) in the housing area decreased likelihood of shedding. This organism has also been found on the inside of the nipple of bottles used to feed calves (ER Atwill, personal communication, 2007). This latter finding would justify keeping separate feeding supplies for calves less than 5-days old from those used for older calves to decrease exposure among young calves. The older the calf is at the time of exposure, the milder their infection will be in general. Dry, clean individual calf housing away from cows and free of moisture with good drainage can decrease exposure to

Cryptosporidium. Exposure of the organism to summer heat and winter cold should decrease the environmental burden of organisms on a farm.

C parvum is the most common calf diarrhea pathogen to be associated with zoonotic disease, most often in veterinary students and those working with affected calves during necropsy, treatment, or clinical examination. Fomites on human clothing, hands, and footwear may transfer the parasite to other calves, pets, or family members when work clothing or footwear are worn home (Pat Blanchard, unpublished observation). Fortunately, most infections are self-limiting in immune competent humans and animals but they may take up to 15 days to resolve.

COCCIDIA

Coccidia in cattle are in the genus *Eimeria* of which *E bovis* and *E zuernii* are the most common and pathogenic.[20] This organism is one of the most common causes of diarrhea in calves from 3- to 6-months old, but infections can be seen in pasture beef calves or group housed calves as young as 3-weeks old. The prepatent period is 15 to 21 days. *Eimeria* can persist in the environment for years so exposure of calves after return from a calf ranch to the home dairy in the absence of a coccidiostat can precipitate the disease. Coccidiosis has not been seen in calf hutch calves (Pat Blanchard, unpublished observation).

Though coccidia can cause severe bloody to watery diarrhea, ill thrift, and rough hair coats, up to 95% of infections are subclinical. Gross lesions may include frank thick blood in the spiral and/or descending colon, red watery contents, and roughened, granular, reddened colon mucosa with petechial hemorrhages and edema of the wall. The gamonts and oocysts of *E bovis* and *E zuernii* form in the crypt cells of the cecum and colon, which then undergo necrosis. Therefore, it is imperative to obtain content from the colon or rectum for parasite testing on necropsy cases because the small intestine content will not contain oocysts. Fresh and fixed cecum and colon sections are valuable because severe infections may have only small numbers of oocysts detectable in the feces but will have classic histologic lesions in the large intestine.

A quick field test for coccidia can be done at necropsy by scraping the abnormal-looking colon mucosa and mixing with a small drop of water on a slide and examining at 200× (combined ocular power of 10× and objective of 20×) magnification to detect oocysts. They will often be present in very large number. Standard detection methods include fecal flotation and McMaster's fecal examination. Feces from multiple animals should be submitted because, later in the infection cycle, very few oocysts may be found despite considerable damage to the large intestine. These animals may become chronic poor doers.

OTHER PARASITES

Abomasal (*Haemonchus, Ostertagia, Trichostrongylus*) and intestinal (*Nematodirus, Trichuris,* and *Oesophagostomum*), parasites generally have prepatent periods greater than 5 weeks and are uncommon causes of diarrhea in calves less than 3-months old. The detection methods include fecal flotation and McMaster's examination.

Giardia duodenalis (also known as *G lamblia* and *G intestinalis*) has been reported to colonize 100% of dairy and beef calves in the first 5-months of life.[32–34] Peak infection rates (85%) and number of cysts shed[34] occur at 5-weeks old and the mean age of first shedding is 30-days old with a prepatent period of 7 to 8 days.[33,34] Because the organism is commonly found in healthy calves and, less often, cows on pasture, particularly periparturient cows, its significance as a causative agent of diarrhea in calves is uncertain and infections are usually subclinical. The organism can colonize the small intestine by attachment to epithelial cells via an adhesive disk but this colonization is extremely rare to find on histopathology (Pat Blanchard, unpublished observation) in calves with diarrhea. Reportedly, it can cause villus atrophy, lymphocytic inflammation, and decreased digestion of nutrients.[32] The organism can remain viable for months in cool, moist environments. *Giardia* can be detected in feces by zinc sulfate or sugar centrifugation type of flotation methods, antigen ELISA, PCR, and FA techniques. Reinfection has been reported to occur rapidly after treatment.[32]

ROTAVIRUS AND CORONAVIRUS

These viruses can be detected in calves as young as 1-day old and most often cause diarrhea in 2- to 24-day old calves, though older naïve calves can also be affected by either virus. Rotavirus has a prepatent period of 1 to 3 days and diarrhea lasts 2 to 5 days if uncomplicated.[2,13] Coronavirus has a prepatent period of 2 days and diarrhea lasts 3 to 6 days after onset.[13] Both viruses are ubiquitous and published reports have varied in whether there is a significant difference between diarrheic and age-matched controls for the presence of either virus. Rotavirus is the most common or second-most common enteric pathogen found in the feces of diarrheic calves, whereas coronavirus is the third-most commonly reported pathogen in numerous surveys.[4–6,15] When examining only calves from necropsies, the authors found coronavirus to be the second-most common pathogen and rotavirus the third (see **Table 3**). This probably reflects more severe disease caused by coronavirus resulting in death of calves compared with rotavirus infections; although multiple pathogens were commonly found with both agents.

Both rotavirus and coronavirus cause villus atrophy, which results in diarrhea due to maldigestion and malabsorption. Maldigestion results in undigested feed in the colon, which leads to bacterial overgrowth and osmotic pressure exacerbating the diarrhea.[13,35] Coronavirus affects a larger portion of the small intestinal villus epithelium and rarely the crypts and often causes colon crypt and adjacent lamina propria histiocyte necrosis; therefore, this virus is more likely than rotavirus to cause severe diarrhea.[13,35] Rotavirus usually affects the caudal small intestine but, in younger calves, has been reported to be more widespread in distribution.[20] Coronavirus affects the proximal small intestine initially, progressing distally and diarrhea onset begins when epithelial cells become infected before the onset of necrosis.[13] Gross lesions of coronavirus in the colon may vary from normal mucosa with diarrhea to lesions similar to those described earlier for attaching and effacing *E coli*. Gross lesions in the small intestine for both viruses are often not detected. Both viruses can be shed by cows in the periparturient period increasing potential exposure of their calves.[20,35] Coronavirus is also more likely to be shed by cows and survives better in the environment in winter months.[35]

Various detection methods exist for both viruses with wide variation in the level of agreement found between methods in several studies. Methods for both viruses include PCR, EM, ELISA, immune-chromatography, lateral-flow antigen capture, FA, isolation, immune-electron microscopy (IEM); and, for rotavirus alone, agglutination and electrophoresis (PAGE).

For rotavirus, agreement between ELISA and EM ranges from 85% to 96% on diagnostic samples[1,4,36,37] and 100% on samples from experimental challenge.[37] However, some commercial ELISA kits have shown a lower sensitivity (78%) and specificity (68%) on diagnostic samples.[2] Agreement between reverse transcription PCR (RT-PCR) and ELISA and RT-PCR and lateral-flow antigen capture on experimental exposed calves was reported as 95% and 85%, respectively.[2] For coronavirus, ELISA methods compared with EM have been reported to have an overall agreement of 88% to 96% in diagnostic samples from diarrhea calves.[4,37,38]

PCR methods, which are increasingly offered by diagnostic laboratories, have a better sensitivity than currently available antigen detection or EM methods for both viruses.[1] Electron microscopy has been reported to detect oral vaccines up to 3 days for rotavirus and 7 days for coronavirus by PCR[1] but Theil and McCloskey[39] found rotavirus in only 1 of 41 serial fecal samples collected from three gnotobiotic calves following oral vaccination. The positive sample was found on day 3 after vaccination and no efforts were made to identify coronavirus in the study. Frequency and duration of PCR detection of oral vaccines has not yet been reported, but it is reasonable to assume that if they can be detected by EM, they would be detectable by PCR.

Some of the variation in agreement between methods is explained by ELISA methods, whether commercial or in-house developed, that may use different antibodies to the virus of interest, resulting in different sensitivity and specificity. Studies by Reynolds and colleagues[37] demonstrated a decreasing percent of agreement for coronavirus between EM and ELISA using samples taken from experimental calves (100%), field surveys (95%), and routine diagnostic submissions (82%). Athanassious and colleagues[4] demonstrated 95% to 96% agreement between rotavirus and coronavirus ELISA and EM methods in diarrhea calves. In their study, fecal samples were collected within 5 to 6 hours after onset of clinical signs and intestinal tissues within 2 days of onset and all samples were frozen at -70°C until tested. Kapil and colleagues[40] reported a marked drop in virus shedding in calves 3-days postinfection with coronavirus. These three studies indicate timing of sampling after onset of diarrhea and quality and storage of samples have an impact on results.

In the Reynolds and colleagues study,[37] rotavirus had a lower agreement between EM and ELISA on field survey samples than diagnostic samples, which might reflect calves with group B rotavirus among survey samples. Group A rotaviruses cause approximately 95% of rotavirus infections in calves and are the predominant type seen in humans; therefore, diagnostic antigen-detection methods (ELISA, lateral-flow, and agglutination) are designed to only detect group A viruses.[1,2] However, group B rotavirus have been reported in calves with diarrhea[41] and can be detected by EM. By EM, these viruses are not distinguishable from group A rotavirus.

FA tests are not as reliable on small intestine for either virus because the infected villus tip cells undergo necrosis and slough. This, combined with postmortem loss of infected epithelial cells, leads to false negative results. One study[36] using small intestine for rotavirus FA noted a 33% agreement between FA and EM. For coronavirus, comparing FA and IHC to direct EM was reported to have a relative sensitivity of 63% to 80%[38,42] and 83%,[42] respectively. For coronavirus, the spiral colon is a more reliable site for FA because the infected cells are retained in the crypts, less susceptible to postmortem loss, and have been reported to persist in the colon longest.[40] Extensive FA positive staining may occur in the spiral colon in early infections because diarrhea onset precedes necrosis of colon cells. Later stage infections, when only rare necrotic crypts surrounded by fibrous tissue are present, will occasionally have focal positive staining. Detection of coronavirus by FA on frozen colon tissue has a good correlation with the presence of colon lesions by histopathology (Pat Blanchard, personal observation).

EM is more reliable for rotavirus, which is stable, shed in large amounts during diarrhea phase, and has a unique size and appearance compared with coronavirus, which is less stable, often appears pleomorphic, and cell membranes and other cell substances may mimic the pleomorphic appearance, causing both false negative and false positive findings.[4] This problem is partially overcome by the experience of the electron microscopist and the storage, freshness, and preparation of the sample. Immunoelectron microscopy eliminates the false positive results but is rarely performed in most diagnostic laboratories. PAGE patterns of rotavirus isolates will allow determination of the group present.[41]

Colostral antibodies help protect against infection following vaccination of dry cows. Oral vaccines with attenuated viruses are available for use in newborn calves. In some cases, the use of both dry cow vaccine and oral calf vaccine seems to negate the positive effect of either alone because the oral vaccine virus binds to colostral antibody, reducing the antibody available for absorption or the virus available for local immunity stimulation.

BVDV

Most BVDv infections in calves less than 30-days old are probably persistent infections. In this age group, BVDv causes a very mild neutrophilic exudate in the crypts of the ileum. This is a nonspecific lesion. BVDv fluorescent antibody testing often reveals widespread staining of smooth muscle and epithelium in the intestine of affected calves. The virus may contribute to diarrhea through nonspecific suppression of the immune system. At CAHFS-Tulare, over the past 10 years, 1.3% of calves submitted for calf diarrhea work up were infected with BVDv. BVDv persistently infected calves may have a higher death loss at a young age when challenged with other enteric pathogens.

The more typical lesions of BVDv, including oral and esophageal ulcers, necrosis of the rumen, and intestine crypt epithelium and Peyer patch lymphocytes are usually seen in cattle between 4- to 14-months old. Colostral antibodies drop to undetectable levels between 4- to 8-months old, so calves become susceptible at that time. Most cattle will have asymptomatic exposures and develop antibodies. A few will become ill (anorexia, fever, diarrhea) but usually recover if no concurrent diseases occur.

OTHER VIRUSES

Torovirus has been documented to be the sole pathogen or the one most consistently present in some calf diarrhea outbreaks in the Midwest.[43] Most positive animals were less than 3-weeks old. The organism can cause small intestine villus atrophy affecting the middle portion of the villi and crypts in the small intestine and colon. The incubation period is 1 to 3 days with diarrhea lasting from 3 to 5 days. *Torovirus* has been detected in cattle from a few days to 10-months old. The virus can be detected by EM but, like coronavirus, the amount of virus shed and a somewhat pleomorphic appearance limit the usefulness of this procedure. Methods to concentrate the virus for improved detection include use of IEM, PCR, and antigen-detection ELISA none of which are widely used outside of research facilities. Serologic surveys of cattle suggest that virus exposure is widespread.

ABOMASITIS AND ABOMASAL BLOAT

Clostridium spp abomasitis occurs in calves less than 7-days old. Gross pathology findings include marked hemorrhage and emphysema of the abomasal wall with gas distention and bloody abomasal content.[20,44] Lesions may extend to involve the rumen, omasum, and reticulum.

Another cause of abomasal bloat, sometimes resulting in rupture, is a gas bloat condition associated with the presence of *Sarcina*, a gram-positive anaerobic cocci found in the soil. The abomasum wall is commonly emphysematous and may have patchy edema, congestion, hemorrhage, or brown to black discoloration from digested blood. *Sarcina* forms packets of 8 to 16 cocci detectable by histopathology in the abomasal lumen and sometimes the wall of affected calves.[45] Studies with this organism alone or in combination with *C perfringens* failed to reproduce the bloat condition (Ken Mills, PhD, Laramie, WY, personal communication, 2006). The appearance of the organism in the abomasum on histopathology is associated with bloat and has not been found in calves (Pat Blanchard, unpublished observation) or goats[46] that die from other causes. Affected calves are less than 30-days old and receive some type of milk product including whole milk or milk replacers and may even be nursing cows on pasture. Esophageal intubation is not effective in relieving the bloat because the tube does not reach the abomasum. Using a large-bore needle inserted in the right flank may relieve the gas. Neither of these abomasal bloat conditions is associated with diarrhea in calves.

NUTRITIONAL-ASSOCIATED CAUSE
Yeast or Fungi

Heavy or prolonged use of antibiotics for treatment or as a component of medicated milk replacers can disrupt normal forestomach and intestinal flora allowing overgrowth of yeast and fungi causing white plaques or adherent curd-like lesions on the mucosa of the rumen, reticulum, and omasum, as well as inflammation in the abomasum. True fungi, such as zygomycetes, can also overgrow and invade the mucosa causing vascular thrombosis of the submucosa with round red-rimmed foci of necrosis in any of the forestomachs, but most often in the abomasum, of calves less than 30-days old. Yeast overgrowth may be profound enough to be found at all levels of the intestine and suggests dysbacteriosis, which may be associated with diarrhea.

Milk Replacer Quality

Osmotic diarrhea can result from poorly digestible milk replacers, which lead to an excess of undigested nutrients in the lower intestine. This can also provide a substrate for bacterial overgrowth and contribute to the diarrhea. Testing of milk replacers to validate the label claims may lead to detection of higher fiber than noted on the label, which would indicate poorly digestible plant proteins may have been substituted for casein, blood-based, or processed soy proteins.[20] The plant proteins, other than processed soy, are generally poorly digestible in nonruminating young calves.

Rumen Acidosis

Rumen acidosis is a common cause of diarrhea in transition cows but not commonly seen in calves less than 3-months old. However, it should be considered if there is evidence of a sudden change in the feed components or sudden access to a high carbohydrate source to which the calf is not conditioned. This can occur when unweaned beef calves are removed from pasture and given grain for the first time. Other events, such as keeping a pen of calves off feed for a prolonged period while processing or vaccinating them, then allowing free-choice access to a day's worth of grain, might lead to rapid consumption by aggressive eaters.

Molybdenosis or Copper Deficiency

This condition is more common in beef calves on pasture because most dairy cow diets are supplemented with copper when molybdenum is high in the diet. There are no specific gross or histologic lesions in the intestine with this condition, but calves may be experiencing concurrent fading of coat color particularly around the eyes, ill-thrift, poor hair quality, and diarrhea. Serum can be tested for copper levels on live calves and cows or liver on dead animals.

SUMMARY

Calf diarrhea is a multifactorial disease related to a combination of host and pathogen factors. The most common pathogens found in diarrheic calves are *Cryptosporidium*, rotavirus, coronavirus, *Salmonella*, attaching and effacing *E coli* (EHEC, EPEC, STEC), and F5 (K99) *E coli*. Increased mortality and morbidity are often due to the presence of more than one pathogen. This article includes a discussion of key information to obtain in a clinical history, the pathogens, pathology findings, and diagnostic methods.

REFERENCES

1. Cho YI, Kim WI, Liu S, et al. Development of a panel of multiplex real-time poly-merase chain reaction assays for simultaneous detection of major agents causing calf diarrhea in feces. J Vet Diagn Invest 2010;22:509–17.
2. Maes RK, Grooms DL, Wise AG, et al. Evaluation of a human group A rotavirus assay for on-site detection of bovine rotavirus. J Clin Microbiol 2003;41:290–4.
3. Eriksson E, Aspan A. Comparison of culture, ELISA and PCR techniques for *Salmonella* detection in faecal samples for cattle, pig and poultry. BMC Vet Res 2007;22:3–21.
4. Athanassious R, Marsolais G, Assaf R, et al. Detection of bovine coronavirus and type A rotavirus in neonatal calf diarrhea and winter dysentery of cattle in Quebec: evaluation of three diagnostic methods. Can Vet J 1994;35:163–9.
5. Izzo MM, Kirkland PD, Mohler VL. Prevalence of major enteric pathogens in Australian dairy calves with diarrhea. Aust Vet J 2011;89:167–73.
6. Naciri M, Lefay MP, Mancassola R, et al. Role of *Cryptosporidium parvum* as a pathogen in neonatal diarrhoea complex in suckling and dairy calves in France. Vet Parasitol 1999;85:245–57.
7. Hammitt MC, Bueschel DM, Keel MK, et al. A possible role of *Clostridium difficile* in the etiology of calf enteritis. Vet Microbiol 2008;127:343–52.
8. Moxley RA, Smith DJ. Attaching-effacing *E. coli* infections in cattle. Vet Clin North Am Food Anim Pract 2010;26(1):29–56.
9. Shaw DJ, Jenkins C, Pearce MC, et al. Shedding patterns of verocytotoxin-producing *Escherichia coli* strains in a cohort of calves and their dams on a Scottish beef farm. Appl Environ Microbiol 2004;70:7456–65.
10. Janke BH, Francis DH, Collins JE, et al. Attaching and effacing *Escherichia coli* infection as a cause of diarrhea in young calves. J Am Vet Med Assoc 1990; 196:897–901.
11. Blanchard P, DeBey B, Akins J, et al. Attaching and effacing E. coli in calves [abstract 29]. In: Program abstracts of the 37th annual meeting of the American Association of Veterinary Laboratory Diagnosticians. Grand Rapids (MI): 1994, p. 29.
12. Janke BH, Francis DH, Collins JE, et al. Attaching and effacing *Escherichia coli* infections in calves, pigs, lambs, and dogs. J Vet Diagn Invest 1989;1:6–11.
13. Foster DM, Smith GW. Pathophysiology of diarrhea in calves. Vet Clin North Am Food Anim Pract 2009;25(1):13–36.

14. Runnels PL, Moon HW, Schneider RA. Development of resistance with host age to adhesion of K99 *Escherichia coli* to isolated intestinal epithelial cells. Infect Immun 1980;28:298–300.
15. de la Fuente R, Garcia A, Ruiz-Santa-Quiteria J, et al. Proportional morbidity rates of enteropathogens among diarrheic dairy calves in central Spain. Prev Vet Med 1998;36:142–5.
16. Cummings KJ, Warnick LD, Alexander KA, et al. The incidence of salmonellosis among dairy herds in the northeastern United States. J Dairy Sci 2009;92: 3766–74.
17. Berge AC, Moore DA, Sischo WM. Prevalence and antimicrobial resistance patterns of *Salmonella* enterica in preweaned calves from dairies and calf ranches. Am J Vet Res 2006;67:1580–8.
18. Anderson RJ, House JK, Smith BP, et al. Epidemiologic and biologic characteristics of salmonellosis on three dairy farms. J Am Vet Med Assoc 2001;219:310–22.
19. Fossler CJ, Wells SW, Kaneene JB, et al. Herd-level factors associated with isolation of *Salmonella* in a multi-state study of conventional and organic dairy farms II. *Salmonella* shedding in calves. Prev Vet Med 2005;70:279–91.
20. Gunn AA, Naylor JA, House JK. Diarrhea. In manifestations and management of disease in neonatal ruminants. In: Smith BP, editor. Large animal internal medicine. 4th edition. St. Louis, MO: Mosby Elsevier; 2009. p. 340–62.
21. Fayer R, Santín M, Xiao L. *Cryptosporidium bovis* n. sp. (*Apicomplexa: Cryptosporidiidae*) in cattle (*Bos taurus*). J Parasitol 2005;91:624–9.
22. Fayer R, Santín M, Trout JM. *Cryptosporidium ryanae* n. sp. (*Apicomplexa: Cryptosporidiidae*) in cattle (*Bos taurus*). Vet Parasitol 2008;156:191–8.
23. Santin M, Trout JM, Xiao L, et al. Prevalence and age-related variation of *Cryptosporidium* species and genotypes in dairy calves. Vet Parasitol 2004;122:103–17.
24. Silverlas C, Naslund K, Bjorkman C, et al. Molecular characterisation of *Cryptosporidium* isolates from Swedish dairy cattle in relation to age, diarrhoea and region. Vet Parasitol 2010;169:289–95.
25. Atwill ER, Harp JA, Jones T, et al. Evaluation of periparturient dairy cows and contact surfaces as a reservoir of *Cryptosporidium parvum* for calfhood infection. Am J Vet Res 1998;59:1116–21.
26. de la Fuente R, Luzon M, Ruiz-Santa-Quiteria JA, et al. *Cryptosporidium* and other concurrent major enteropathogens in 1 to 30-day-old diarrheic dairy calves in central Spain. Vet Parasitol 1999;80:179–85.
27. Trotz-Williams LA, Martin SW, Leslie KE, et al. Calf-level risk factors for neonatal diarrhea and shedding of *Cryptosporidium parvum* in Ontario dairy calves. Prev Vet Med 2007;82:12–28.
28. Peng X, Murphy T, Holden NM. Evaluation of the effect of temperature on the die-off rate for *Cryptosporidium parvum* oocysts in water, soils, and feces. Appl Environ Microbiol 2008;74:7101–7.
29. Jenkins MB, Bowman DD, Fogarty EA, et al. *Cryptosporidium parvum* oocyst inactivation in three soil types at various temperatures and water potentials. Soil Biol Biochem 2002;34:1101–9.
30. Li X, Atwill ER, Dunbar LA, et al. Seasonal temperature fluctuations induces rapid inactivation of *Cryptosporidium parvum*. Environ Sci Technol 2005;39:4484–9.
31. Szonyi B, Chang YF, Wade SE, et al. Evaluation of factors associated with the risk of infection with *Cryptosporidium parvum* in dairy calves. Am J Vet Res 2012;73: 76–85.
32. O'Handley RM, Olson ME. Giardiasis and cryptosporidiosis in ruminant. Vet Clin North Am Food Anim Pract 2006;22:623–43.

33. O'Handley RM, Cockwill C, McAllister TA, et al. Duration of naturally acquired giardiosis and cryptosporidiosis in dairy calves and their association with diarrhea. J Am Vet Med Assoc 1999;214:391–6.
34. Ralston BJ, McAllister TA, Olson MA. Prevalence and infection pattern of naturally acquired giardiasis and cryptosporidiosis in range beef calves and their dams. Vet Parasitol 2003;114:113–22.
35. Boileau MJ, Kapil S. Bovine coronavirus associated syndromes. Vet Clin North Am Food Anim Pract 2010;26:123–46.
36. Benfield DA, Stotz IJ, Nelson EA, et al. Comparison of a commercial enzyme-linked immunosorbent assay with electron microscopy, fluorescent antibody, and virus isolation for the detection of bovine and porcine rotavirus. Am J Vet Res 1984;45:1998–2002.
37. Reynolds DJ, Chasey D, Scott AC, et al. Evaluation of ELISA and electron microscopy for the detection of coronavirus and rotavirus in bovine faeces. Vet Rec 1984;114:397–401.
38. Tahir RA, Pomeroy KA, Goyal SM. Evaluation of shell vial cell culture technique for the detection of bovine coronavirus. J Vet Diagn Invest 1995;7:301–4.
39. Theil KW, McCloskey CM. Rotavirus shedding in feces of gnotobiotic calves orally inoculated with a commercial rotavirus-coronavirus vaccine. J Vet Diagn Invest 1995;7:427–32.
40. Kapil S, Trent AM, Goyal SM. Excretion and persistence of bovine coronavirus in neonatal calves. Arch Virol 1990;115:127–32.
41. Chang KO, Parwani AV, Smith D, et al. Detection of group B rotaviruses in fecal samples from diarrheic calves and adult cows and characterization of their VP7 genes. J Clin Microbiol 1997;35:2107–10.
42. Dar AM, Kapil S, Goyal SM. Comparison of immunohistochemistry, electron microscopy, and direct fluorescent antibody test for the detection of bovine coronavirus. J Vet Diagn Invest 1998;10:152–7.
43. Hoet AE, Paul R, Nielsen PR, et al. Detection of bovine torovirus and other enteric pathogens in feces from diarrhea cases in cattle. J Vet Diagn Invest 2003;15:205–12.
44. Van Kruiningen HJ, Nyaoke CA, Sidor IF, et al. Clostridial abomasal disease in Connecticut dairy calves. Can Vet J 2009;50:857–60.
45. Edwards GT, Woodger NG, Barlow AM, et al. *Sarcina*-like bacteria associated with bloat in young lambs and calves. Vet Rec 2008;163:391–3.
46. DeBey BM, Blanchard PC, Durfee PT. Abomasal bloat associated with *Sarcina*-like bacteria in goat kids. J Am Vet Med Assoc 1996;209:1468–9.

Field Disease Diagnostic Investigation of Neonatal Calf Diarrhea

David R. Smith, DVM, PhD

KEYWORDS

- Calf • Diarrhea • Epidemiology • Outbreak • Investigation • Diagnostics

KEY POINTS

- Diarrhea is a leading cause of sickness and death of beef and dairy calves in their first month of life.
- Field investigations of outbreaks of neonatal calf diarrhea should be conducted for the purposes of (1) reducing the losses associated with existing cases and (2) preventing new cases from occurring.
- Veterinarians investigating outbreaks of neonatal calf diarrhea must first make recommendations for treating affected calves and then take action to protect susceptible and unborn calves from ongoing illness.
- Knowing the etiologic agent may provide an explanation for the proximal cause of a calf's illness or death, but that knowledge rarely explains the outbreak or provides a solution for treatment, control, or prevention.
- The goal is to conduct a useful outbreak investigation—one that leads to a solution to the problem.

INTRODUCTION

One of the most likely reasons for young beef or dairy calves to become sick or die is diarrhea.[1] The disease is a detriment to calf health and well-being.[2,3] Also, neonatal calf diarrhea can be economically important to cattle producers because of poor calf performance, death, and the expense of medications and labor to treat sick calves. The act of catching and treating young calves puts farmers and ranchers at risk of physical injury by the calf or dam, and many producers are disheartened by seeing calves become sick or die at only 1 or 2 weeks of age. Finally, there may be public health risks associated with some outbreaks of neonatal calf diarrhea because (1) some diarrhea

The author has nothing to disclose.
Department of Pathobiology and Population Medicine, College of Veterinary Medicine, PO Box 6100, Mississippi State, MS 39762, USA
E-mail address: dsmith@cvm.msstate.edu

pathogens of calves also make people sick and (2) an important reason for using anti-biotics on many beef and dairy farms is to treat young calves for diarrhea.

Until a serious outbreak occurs, veterinarians may not be aware that cattle producers are dealing with neonatal calf diarrhea problems. Veterinarians investi-gating outbreaks of neonatal calf diarrhea must first make recommendations for treat-ing affected calves and then take action to protect susceptible and unborn calves from ongoing illness. Finally, attention should focus on determining what future actions might prevent the disease in subsequent calving periods or seasons.[4] Although knowl-edge of the pathogens involved is often useful information, outbreak investigations sometimes become sidetracked in the sole pursuit of an etiologic agent rather than identifying more useful explanations for the outbreak. Knowing the etiologic agent may provide an explanation for the proximal cause of a calf's illness or death, but that knowledge rarely explains the outbreak or provides a solution for treatment, control, or prevention. The goal, then, is to conduct a useful outbreak investiga-tion—one that leads to a solution to the problem.

PRINCIPLES OF DISEASE OUTBREAK INVESTIGATION

Veterinarians are often asked to investigate outbreaks of animal death or disease, including those related to neonatal calf diarrhea. The objectives of these investigations are commonly to (1) reduce the losses associated with existing cases and (2) prevent new cases from occurring. These objectives are met by (1) confirming the clinical diag-nosis so that affected individuals are treated appropriately, (2) making an appropriate population diagnosis to determine the reasons for the outbreak, (3) identifying actions that can be taken to prevent new cases or future outbreaks, and (4) effectively commu-nicating the plan of action. It can be difficult to provide solutions to disease outbreaks, but success is more likely if an organized, epidemiologic approach to outbreak inves-tigation is followed.[5,6]

Disease outbreaks (epidemics) are typically defined as an unexpected increase in disease or death, typically occurring during a brief period of time. Outbreaks may occur because of a common (point-source) exposure (eg, the potato salad at the church picnic). These types of outbreaks are typically rapid in development and reso-lution or they may become propagated epidemics (eg, you got sick from the church supper and then your family got sick and passed it on to friends at school). Propagated epidemics are typically characterized by less rapid but ongoing transmission from animal to animal. The distinction between these two types of outbreaks sometimes becomes blurred, but often they are distinguishable by observing the epidemic curve. Methods to prevent new cases may differ depending on the type of epidemic (eg, removing the potato salad or isolating sick individuals).[7]

Outbreak investigations involve an orderly process to characterize the outbreak:

- Interview key individuals (eg, owners, caretakers, veterinarians, nutritionists, and other stakeholders)
- Verify the clinical diagnosis and assure that treatments are appropriate
- Identify the factors responsible for the outbreak: make a population diagnosis
  - Establish a system for collecting information
  - Define what a case is and what a case is not
  - Define the population at risk
  - Characterize the outbreak by time, space, and unit (animal, pen, herd, region)
  - Determine the nature of the outbreak (point source, propagated)
  - Develop hypotheses about possible causal factors
  - Test hypotheses using epidemiologic principles

- Develop strategies to prevent new cases and future outbreaks
  - Identify control points and corrective actions based on the knowledge of causal factors and key determinants
- Communicate observations and recommendations with the key individuals
  - Validate that recommendations are being performed
  - Monitor progress

INVESTIGATING OUTBREAKS OF NEONATAL CALF DIARRHEA

Identify the key individuals early in the course of the investigation. Although you may be reporting to the owner, other individuals may be able to provide history or other details unknown to the owner. Key individuals include those with direct financial interests (eg, the owner); employee caretakers who may know the most about day-to-day care and practice; and other parties, such as other veterinarians, nutritional consultants, or other advisors that may have special knowledge of the circumstances. Capture names and contact information at the start of the investigation.

Verify the Diagnosis and Assure that Treatments are Appropriate

Early in the outbreak investigation it is vital to conduct at least a preliminary examination of affected animals. This process includes a walk-through of the herd and facilities, completing physical examinations or postmortem examinations, and submitting samples to the diagnostic laboratory (see article by Blanchard in this issue) to verify the clinical diagnosis.[5,8] Assure that affected calves are receiving medically appropriate treatment, so that ongoing losses are minimized while the outbreak is being investigated. Determine through history and records analysis that this is indeed an outbreak (defined as an increased incidence of disease compared with expected or historical rates). Sometimes an outbreak is really a sudden awareness on the owner's or caretaker's part of a disease process that has been ongoing for some time.

Identify the Factors Responsible for the Outbreak: Make a Population Diagnosis

Establish a system for recording information

Few cow-calf and dairy operations collect animal health data in a format that is easily analyzed. If records exist at all, they may be on paper (eg, in pocket-sized ranch books) or in an electronic format with free text fields, none of which allow the veterinarian or the producer to quickly and easily discover animal health relationships. Some electronic record-keeping systems capture health information and may present information in standard graphs or summaries, but do not allow easy querying of health relationships. Free text fields are difficult or impossible to analyze because of misspelled words, multiple names, or descriptors for the same disease (eg, diarrhea, scours, loose, enteric) and multiple pieces of information in the same field (eg, scours, T103.8, bolus and fluids, retreat afternoon, watch out for the cow). The lack of a simple record-keeping system has hindered many disease outbreak investigations. It simply becomes too costly to wade through inefficient record systems to get the needed information from which questions can be asked. A desirable system for investigating neonatal calf diarrhea is one that captures individual calf information for all calves at risk, not just affected calves. Useful information includes the calf's identification, the identification of the dam, the age of the dam, the calf's birth date, the date of onset of the illness, the date of onset of other illnesses, and information describing various risk factors of interest.

Define a case

A critical, but too often ignored, component of any disease outbreak investigation is specifying what a case is and what it is not. Neonatal calf diarrhea is no exception.

Diarrhea is a subjective diagnosis and accompanying clinical signs (eg, dehydration, fever, and level of depression) may or may not be relevant to the specific syndrome associated with the outbreak of interest. For example, the complaint may be about high mortality in calves developing diarrhea at 1 to 3 weeks' of age. So, do you count as cases calves with fever or dehydration but no observed diarrhea? What about calves with diarrhea at 60 days' of age or calves with distended abdomens and pasty stools? The definition of a case is not always obvious but it is important. Having a reasonable level of specificity in the case definition is necessary to avoid the confusion of looking for a single solution to more than one problem. However, overspecifying the case definition may cause confusion because only part of the problem is being investigated.

Define the population at risk

Incidence is a measure of the driving force of disease: the rate at which new cases of disease are occurring. The population at risk is the denominator for incidence and by itself is a measure of importance because it may describe a dynamic population. The process of gathering history, conducting physical examinations, reviewing the literature, and developing a case definition should help clarify who is at risk for the disease. Only a subset of animals in a population may be at risk for a given disease based on various conditions or characteristics, including age, gender, breed, physical location, and so forth (eg, only females are at risk for pregnancy and only pregnant cows are at risk for abortion). Neonatal calf diarrhea typically occurs at a narrow range in age, so, for example, it may be appropriate to define the population at risk as calves less than 4 weeks' of age (**Fig. 1**).

Characterize the outbreak by time, space, and unit (eg, animal, pen, or herd)

Often a disease outbreak investigation is initiated long after cases have occurred. It may be possible to reconstruct the outbreak by asking questions, analyzing health records, or preferably both. The most common way of doing this would be to characterize the outbreak by who got sick, when, and where. The *who* may be specifically identified individuals about whom you may have additional information or it may be group-level information (eg, the pens or groups that have been affected). This process may be iterative because there may be refinements in the case definition and the

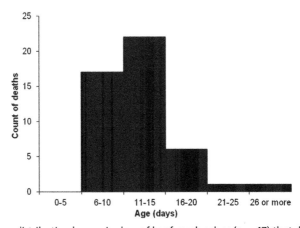

Fig. 1. Frequency distribution by age in days of beef ranch calves (n = 47) that died of neonatal calf diarrhea among a population of 402 calves. (*From* Smith DR, Grotelueschen DM, Knott T, et al. Population dynamics of undifferentiated neonatal calf diarrhea among ranch beef calves. Bovine Practitioner 2008;42(8):1–8; with permission.)

definition of the population at risk as the outbreak is reconstructed. It may be useful to graphically portray this information, for example, in the form of frequency histograms. A frequency histogram of particular interest is the count of cases plotted by time, also known as an epidemic curve (**Fig. 2**).

Determine the nature of the outbreak

The shape of the epidemic curve may provide clues about the nature of the disease process and factors that have favored the occurrence of clinical signs.[7] For example, outbreaks that occur as a point-source epidemic (eg, because of a sudden exposure to a pathogen, the sudden loss of immunity, or something that suddenly facilitates pathogen transmission) may be evidenced as an epidemic curve with a high peak in a relatively short period of time. When the outbreak is propagated (eg, when the disease process is one of ongoing transmission or there is a continuous presence of risk factors), the epidemic curve may appear flatter over a longer period of time. Sometimes outbreaks begin as a point-source exposure but are followed by secondary transmission and a propagated epidemic.

Develop hypotheses about possible causal risk factors

The causes of neonatal diarrhea in calves include more than the etiologic agent. In fact, it may be rare that knowledge of the presence of an agent by itself leads to a solution to outbreaks of neonatal calf diarrhea. To make effective recommendations for corrective actions following an outbreak, one often needs to understand how the pathogen interacts within the production system. For example, once you know the agent involved, it might still be useful to understand the various sources of the agent and routes of transmission on the farm.

Neonatal calf diarrhea is a complex, multifactorial, and temporally dynamic disease process.[9–11] The factors that explain neonatal disease are the agent, factors related to host resistance or susceptibility to disease, and factors about the environment that favor the host or agent. These factors interact dynamically over time. To control the disease or prevent its occurrence, it is important to understand the relationships between these multiple factors and how they interact within the production system.[12] It may be more useful to diagnose the failure of passive transfer or recognize a vehicle of pathogen transmission than to know the specific agent involved. Population diagnostics is concerned with correctly diagnosing or classifying the outbreak by agent, host, environment, and temporal factors.

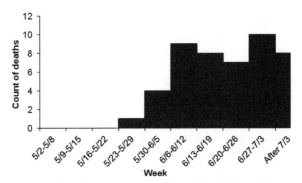

Fig. 2. Epidemic curve of deaths occurring each week of the calving season caused by neonatal calf diarrhea among beef ranch calves. (*From* Smith DR, Grotelueschen DM, Knott T, et al. Population dynamics of undifferentiated neonatal calf diarrhea among ranch beef calves. Bovine Practitioner 2008;42(8):1–8; with permission.)

Agent factors

Numerous infectious agents have been recovered from calves with neonatal diarrhea.[9,10,12–19] The most common agents of neonatal calf diarrhea include bacteria, such as *Escherichia coli* and *Salmonella*; viruses, such as rotavirus and coronavirus; and protozoa, such as cryptosporidia. Bovine rotavirus, bovine coronavirus, and cryptosporidia can be found in most cattle populations and can be recovered from calves in herds not experiencing calf diarrhea.[12] It is not unusual to be able to find multiple agents in herds experiencing outbreaks of calf diarrhea, suggesting that even during outbreaks, more than one agent may be involved. The adult cow herd commonly serves as the reservoir of pathogens from one year to the next.[20–25]

Often outbreak investigations take place long after cases have occurred, so opportunities to identify pathogens have past. If neonatal diarrhea cases are ongoing, pathogen diagnostics may be helpful to the investigation (see article by Blanchard in this issue). For example, it may be useful to know if the pathologic condition is caused by bacterial or viral pathogens because that knowledge may guide treatment decisions, lead to hypotheses about routes and sources of exposure, or create awareness of zoonotic potential. Also, serologic responses or even recovery of the agent are not necessarily clear indications that the pathogen is a primary pathogen in the condition being investigated. The recovery of one pathogen may not mean that there are not other players, and the relative prevalence of agents recovered from neonatal calf diarrhea cases may simply reflect the relative ease of detecting the agent. Finally, diagnostics for the purpose of outbreak investigation are almost always conducted to answer population-based questions. Rarely is the question about what pathogen is causing diarrhea in a particular calf. More often the question is whether to and how to adequately test for pathogens that are affecting the health of the herd.

The investigator might first determine if knowledge of the agents involved will change the way current cases are treated or future cases will be prevented. If it would be useful to know the pathogens involved, it is reasonable to want the testing process to accurately reflect the status of the herd.[26,27] Ineffective herd-level testing might either fail to identify important pathogens present in the herd or falsely classify a herd as having a pathogen it does not, either way, misdirecting the investigation.

To determine if herd-level testing will have adequate negative or positive predictive value you must know: (1) what samples and test methods are appropriate for diagnosing the presence of the pathogens of interest, (2) how well those tests perform, (3) if samples can be collected from representative cases or appropriate environmental sources, (4) if an adequate number of cases can be sampled, and (5) how many test-positive results are necessary to classify the herd as infected. The number of samples needed to make a herd-level diagnosis depends on (1) the expected prevalence of the pathogen within the herd, (2) the performance of the test on individual samples (eg, sensitivity and specificity), and (3) the likelihood of the herd having the pathogen.[26] When a diagnosis is rare, then the herd-level positive predictive value may be low, especially if the herd-level specificity is low. When a diagnosis is common, the herd-level negative predictive value may be low, especially if the herd-level sensitivity is low.

In conducting population (eg, herd-level) diagnostics, the herd is often classified by a process of testing many individuals. In this situation, the herd-level sensitivity improves because of the many opportunities to find the agent; however, the herd-level specificity decreases because there are more opportunities to find a false-positive result. Therefore, confirmatory testing using a test of high specificity (eg, serial testing) may be important.[26] For example, a single bovine viral diarrhea virus (BVDV)-positive enzyme-linked immunosorbent assay test result might lead the investigator to think BVDV is circulating in the herd, taking the investigation and proposed corrective actions down a particular (and possibly costly) path. Confirmatory testing (eg, using immunohistochemistry) might be prudent before going down that path. The issues of predictive value of a test are equally relevant to diagnostics of host, environmental, and temporal risk factors.

Host factors

Calves obtain passive immunity against common agents of calf diarrhea after absorbing antibodies from colostrum or colostrum supplements shortly after birth.[28–30] The quantity of antibodies absorbed is determined by the quality and quantity of colostrum the calf ingests and how soon after birth it is ingested. The presence of maternal antibodies against specific agents in colostrum requires that the dam had prior exposure to antigens of the agent. Vaccines are used to immunize the dam against specific agents, and some commercially available colostrum supplements contain polyclonal or monoclonal antibodies directed against specific agents. Unfortunately, the use of vaccines or colostrum supplements does not always prevent neonatal calf diarrhea.

Calves commonly become ill or die of neonatal diarrhea within 1 to 2 weeks' of age.[9,13,15,31,32] The relatively narrow age range for neonatal calf diarrhea is not explained solely by the incubation period of the agents. Diarrhea may be observed in colostrum-deprived and gnotobiotic calves within a few days of pathogen challenge regardless of age.[33–35] Calves may have an age-specific susceptibility to neonatal diarrhea that occurs as maternal immunity is waning and before the calf is capable of an active immune response.[28]

Regardless of the reason for the age-specificity of neonatal calf diarrhea, this period defines the age of calf susceptibility as well as the age calves are most likely to become infective and shed the agents in their feces.[25,36–40] Age-specificity of susceptibility and infectivity has important implications for preventing the transmission of the pathogens of neonatal diarrhea because, in some calving systems, the number of susceptible and infective calves can change dynamically with time (**Fig. 3**). At times, the number of potentially infective calves may greatly outnumber the number of susceptible calves resulting in an overwhelming opportunity for effective contacts.

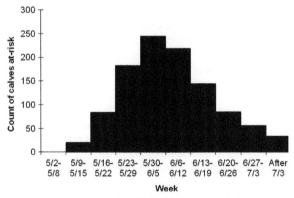

Fig. 3. Frequency distribution of the number of ranch calves considered at risk for neonatal calf diarrhea for each week of the calving season. The at-risk population was defined as the number of calves born in the previous 3 weeks and alive at the beginning of that week. (*From* Smith DR, Grotelueschen DM, Knott T, et al. Population dynamics of undifferentiated neonatal calf diarrhea among ranch beef calves. Bovine Practitioner 2008;42(8):1–8; with permission.)

The dam's age is important to a calf's risk for undifferentiated neonatal diarrhea. Calves born to heifers are at a higher risk for neonatal diarrhea and have lower maternal antibody levels than calves born to older cows.[41] Calves born to heifers are probably more susceptible to disease because, compared with older cows, heifers produce less volume and lower quality of colostrum, may have poorer mothering skills, and are more likely to experience dystocia.[42,43]

Environmental factors

The rate and magnitude of pathogen exposure as well as the ability of the calf to resist disease may be affected by environmental conditions. Exposure to pathogens may occur through direct contact with other cattle or via contact with contaminated environmental surfaces. Environmental hygiene has long been recognized as important for controlling neonatal calf diarrhea,[44,45] but providing effective hygiene has often been a challenge. An effective contact is an exposure to pathogens of a dose load or duration sufficient to cause disease. Crowded conditions increase opportunities for effective contacts with infected animals or contaminated surfaces. Ambient temperature (eg, excessive heat or cold) and moisture (eg, mud or snow) are important stressors that impair the ability of the calf to resist disease and may influence pathogen numbers as well as opportunities for oral ingestion.

Temporal factors

Risk factors related to time can be associated with calendar time (ie, chronologic order [eg, where a factor occurs on the calendar]) or relative time (ie, time measured from a zero point to an event [eg, the time that has elapsed since birth: age]).[32]

Host susceptibility, pathogen exposure, and pathogen transmission occur dynamically over calendar time within the calving season in beef herds and across seasons in dairies.[12] Although the adult cow herd likely serves as the reservoir of neonatal diarrhea pathogens from year to year,[20–25] the average dose load of pathogen exposure to calves is likely to increase over time within a calving season because calves infected earlier serve as pathogen multipliers and become the primary source of exposure to younger susceptible calves. This multiplier effect can result in high calf infectivity and widespread environmental contamination with pathogens.[46] Each calf serves as growth media for pathogen production, amplifying the dose load of the pathogen it received.[35–37] Therefore, calves born later in a calving season may receive larger dose loads of pathogens and, in turn, may become relatively more infective by growing even greater numbers of agents. Eventually, the dose load of pathogens overwhelms the calf's ability to resist disease. These factors alone or in combination may explain observations that calves born later in the calving season are at greater risk for disease or death (**Fig. 4**).[31,32]

Test causal hypotheses using epidemiologic principles

The specific epidemiologic methods used to identify causes for disease outbreak will vary depending on the nature of the outbreak, time and resources available, and how well cases can be identified and exposures quantified. In disease causal theory, each factor that contributes to the development of disease is a component cause. Disease is observed when various component causes add up to complete a sufficient cause, which explains why some component causes are observed in the absence of disease (eg, we might recover *Cryptosporidia* from the feces of calves without diarrhea). This concept also explains why the manager of a herd that does a good job of assuring passive transfer might blame calf diarrhea on bad weather, whereas the manager of a herd in a moderate climate might observe diarrhea when they have been lax about assuring adequate colostrum intake. Removing one component cause means that the

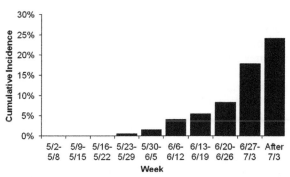

Fig. 4. Cumulative incidence of death caused by neonatal calf diarrhea for each week of the calving season in beef ranch calves. Cumulative incidence was calculated as the number of deaths occurring each week divided by the number of calves at risk for undifferentiated neonatal calf diarrhea. (*From* Smith DR, Grotelueschen DM, Knott T, et al. Population dynamics of undifferentiated neonatal calf diarrhea among ranch beef calves. Bovine Practitioner 2008;42(8):1–8; with permission.)

sufficient cause is not completed and, thus, disease is not observed.[47] For example, one sufficient cause for neonatal calf diarrhea might include component causes of (1) exposure to rotavirus, (2) failure of passive transfer, and (3) weather stress. In the absence of other completed sufficient causes, the removal of any one of these factors would keep calves from developing diarrhea. In general, the objective of the investigation is to determine which possible component causes are contributing to the completion of a sufficient cause and determine which component causes (also known as causal factors or risk factors) are key determinants. Key determinants are those causal factors that can be modified. In the simple example described earlier, we might find it difficult to prevent exposure to rotavirus or correct the weather, so improving passive transfer might be the key determinant.

Gay[48] recently reviewed causal thinking about animal diseases. Koch,[49] Hill,[50] Susser,[51] and Evans[52] have described important causal criteria for health investigations. Each has helped guide our thinking about causes of disease.[48] Each suggests making a case for a causal relationship by finding the proposed cause (1) preceding the effect, (2) having a strong association with the effect, (3) being associated with the effect in more than one study, (4) demonstrating a dose effect, and (5) being consistent with current knowledge. These criteria can help guide the outbreak investigation; although, it is important to recognize that none are necessary or sufficient for determining if a causal relationship exists. Also important is the recognition of the cognitive biases that may prevent veterinarians from drawing the correct conclusions from an investigation.[48]

Sometimes the primary causal question is this: What is different about the calves that got sick and those that did not? But more often the question is this: What is the difference between this herd and other herds not experiencing an outbreak? Some causal factors are characteristics of individuals; other causes are characteristics of groups or herds. If the important causal factors occur at the herd level, it will not be possible to measure this association by comparing (statistically or otherwise) affected and nonaffected calves within a single herd. For example, if an important causal factor is the presence of BVDV circulating among cattle in the herd, it is likely that all calves become exposed to the virus, whether they get sick or not. The inference that BVDV is contributing to disease comes from comparing its presence in this herd with what is expected or observed in other herds. On the other hand, in this same herd, it may be possible to determine that failure of passive protection is also a causal factor by comparing postsuckling immunoglobulin G levels between affected and nonaffected calves within the same herd.

Outbreak investigations of neonatal calf diarrhea are usually qualitative rather than quantitative because useful quantitative data (eg, from health records) are often not available for analysis. A qualitative investigation relies on more subjective observations, including partial records, memory, and perceptions of relationships. Causal inferences in qualitative investigations are largely based on systems of logic developed by John Stuart Mill in the nineteenth century.[48] According to Mill, a causal factor might be identified by the method of agreement if the factor is common to multiple instances of the outcome when other factors are dissimilar (eg, finding that scours outbreaks are common to herds feeding a particular milk replacer, even though other management practices differ). A causal factor might also be identified by the method of difference if a particular factor differs, whereas others remain the same (eg, if calves receiving milk replacer from one bag develop diarrhea, but calves on the same farm receiving milk replacer from another bag do not). Finally, causal relationships may be revealed by the method of concomitant variations if the risk for the outcome changes with the level of the risk factor, all other factors being the same (eg, the more time that calves remain in the maternity pen, the greater the incidence of diarrhea).

When data are available, a quantitative approach is often more useful for discovering causal relationships and evaluating the effectiveness of interventions. The best study design for evaluating causal relationships depends on the circumstances. There are 3 basic observational study designs: (1) case-control, (2) cohort or longitudinal, and (3) cross-sectional. Case-control studies compare odds of exposure among cases to the odds of exposure among noncases. Case-control studies excel when the disease is rare and when there are many potential exposures to test. Cohort and longitudinal studies compare incidence of disease among subjects with an exposure to the incidence of those without the exposure. Cohort and longitudinal studies are best when data exist to follow subjects over time, either prospectively or retrospectively. Cross-sectional studies look at the relationship between disease and exposure prevalence at a point in time.[53]

The statistical measure of association is important because it helps relate the strength of the relationship between the risk factor and the occurrence of disease. When the outcome is dichotomous (eg, diseased or not diseased), the measure of association is the odds ratio or (in some cases) relative risk (RR). These measures are measures of the odds, probability, or incidence rate of observing disease with an exposure level compared with another exposure level (**Figs. 5** and **6**). If the odds ratio has a value of 1, then the exposure is not associated with the disease. If the odds ratio is greater than 1, then that exposure is associated with the disease. If the odds ratio is less than 1, then the exposure is associated with the absence of disease (eg, it is protective from disease). The further the odds ratio is from 1, the stronger the association.

Often quantitative analyses use statistical measures, such as the P value, to help make causal inferences.[54] The P value helps us judge the role of chance in observing the measure of association. It is the probability of observing that relationship, or something more extreme, if in truth no relationship exists. It is a common convention in research to consider a finding statistical significant when the P value is equal to or less than 0.05. However, outbreak investigations often involve small sample sizes with low power to detect differences at that level of significance. In outbreak investigations, it is usually appropriate to interpret the P value liberally, if at all.

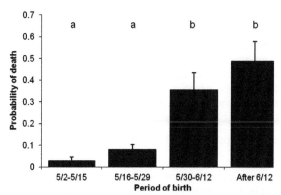

Fig. 5. Model-adjusted probability for calves to die of neonatal calf diarrhea, depending on the period of time the calf was born during the calving season. Calves differed significantly in their risk for death depending on how late in the calving season they were born. Error bars represent the standard error of the mean. The outcomes of variables with different superscripts are statistically different ($P \leq .05$). Compared with calves born in the first 4 weeks, calves born in the last month of calving were 10 times more likely to die (relative risk = 10). (*From* Smith DR, Grotelueschen DM, Knott T, et al. Population dynamics of undifferentiated neonatal calf diarrhea among ranch beef calves. Bovine Practitioner 2008;42(8):1–8; with permission.)

Develop Strategies to Prevent New Cases and Future Outbreaks

With some luck, the result of the outbreak investigation, whether qualitative or quantitative, is a list of potential causal factors that may relate to the agent, host immunity, or the environment. The art of the investigation is determining which factors are key determinants (also called control points) for preventing new cases and future outbreaks of neonatal calf diarrhea. The corrective actions should be (1) manageable (ie, within the capabilities of the caretakers), (2) economical (ie, not cost more than the disease), and (3) most likely to be effective (ie, to have the greatest impact).

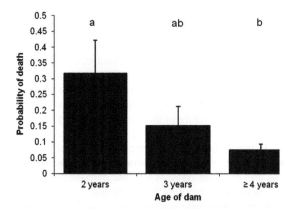

Fig. 6. Model-adjusted probability for calves to die of neonatal calf diarrhea for calves born to dams of different ages. Error bars represent the standard error of the mean. The outcomes of variables with different superscripts are statistically different ($P \leq .05$). Compared with calves born to mature cows, calves born from heifers were 4 times more likely to die (relative risk = 4). (*From* Smith DR, Grotelueschen DM, Knott T, et al. Population dynamics of undifferentiated neonatal calf diarrhea among ranch beef calves. Bovine Practitioner 2008;42(8):1–8; with permission.)

Decisions on the relative importance of various causal factors in the outbreak should include consideration for the impact of the factor on the exposed (attributable risk of exposure) and on the population (population attributable risk). For example, attributable risk of exposure estimates the proportion of cases among the exposed that are actually caused by that exposure. Some calves infected with failure of passive transfer do not develop diarrhea and some develop diarrhea for other reasons, so for calves with failure of passive transfer, what proportion of cases are caused by failure of passive transfer? Attributable risk of exposure is a function of relative risk.

Attributable risk of exposure = (RR-1)/RR

where RR is relative risk.

Not all calves in the population have the causal exposure but they may still develop diarrhea. For example, if failure of passive transfer is suspected as a causal factor in the outbreak, then the impact to the herd (population attributable risk) of taking corrective action to improve passive transfer depends on how strong the association is between failure of passive transfer and diarrhea and how commonly failure of passive transfer occurs.

Population attributable risk $= P_E \times (RR-1)/(P_E \times [RR-1]) + 1)$

where P_E is probability of exposure (to failure of passive transfer) and RR is relative risk (of diarrhea for calves with failure of passive transfer compared to calves with adequate passive transfer).

For this example, the proportion of cases prevented in the herd (population attributable risk) by correcting failure of passive transfer is greater for herds with high rates of failure of passive transfer.

Biocontainment of neonatal calf diarrhea

Biosecurity is the sum of actions taken to prevent introducing a disease agent into a population (pen, herd, region), whereas *biocontainment* describes the actions taken to control or prevent the transmission of a pathogen already present in the population.[55] In the context of disease, the term *control* refers to actions that reduce the prevalence of infected individuals (eg, actions to treat infected individuals to eliminate infection). The term *prevention* refers to actions that reduce the rate of pathogen transmission or disease occurrence (ie, reduce the incidence of new infections).

In theory, neonatal calf diarrhea could be prevented by (1) eliminating the pathogens from the herd and its environment (eg, create a biosecure herd), (2) improving calf resistance to disease, or (3) altering the production system to minimize opportunities for calves to be exposed to existing pathogens and transmitting the infection to others. However, the endemic nature of the common pathogens of neonatal calf diarrhea makes it unlikely that cattle populations could be made biosecure from these agents; therefore, a biocontainment approach to control neonatal calf diarrhea seems prudent and logical.[55,56] Biocontainment actions against neonatal diarrhea might include those that improve passive transfer of maternal antibodies or reducing effective contacts. Maternal immunity is important to calf resistance to enteric agents,[11,57] but maternal immunity wanes with time.[28] Dairy producers might be able to improve maternal immunity by managing colostrum quality and quantity, but managers of extensive beef cattle systems have limited practical opportunities to improve rates of passive antibody transfer. In addition, vaccines are not available against all pathogens of calf diarrhea, may not induce sufficient cross-protection,[40] and pathogens may evade the protection afforded by vaccination by evolving away from vaccine strains.[58]

Effective contacts can be prevented by (1) physically separating animals, (2) reducing the level of exposure (eg, through the use of sanitation or dilution over space), or (3) minimizing contact time. These principles have been successfully applied in calf hutch systems to control neonatal diseases in dairy calves.[59] Various systems for biocontainment have been developed to prevent neonatal calf diarrhea in beef herds.[60–62] Each of these are management strategies to prevent effective contacts by reducing the opportunities for exposure and subsequent transmission. For example, the Sandhills Calving System[63] prevents effective contacts among beef calves by (1) segregating calves by age to prevent direct and indirect transmission of pathogens from older to younger calves and (2) scheduled movement of pregnant cows to clean calving pastures to minimize the pathogen dose load in the environment and minimizing contact time between calves and the larger portion of the cow herd.

Some herds are large enough to conduct their own in-house trials, or multiple herds might be included in a study to test the usefulness of a potential corrective action. If so, it is important to follow a valid experimental design with appropriate methods of data analysis.[64]

Communicate Your Observations and Findings with the Key Individuals

A written report should quickly follow the investigation. In the report, in simple language restate the problem, summarize the findings, explain your interpretation of the findings, and make recommendations to correct the problem. Use graphs, charts, and tables to supplement the report. Consider the risk for subsequent liability and be as complete as possible without overstating your case.

Validate that recommendations are being performed

The corrective actions recommended should be measureable. For example, measurable actions are that pregnant cows move to a new calving pasture every 7 days, calves are removed from the maternity barn within 4 hours of birth, or that 1 gal of colostrum is fed in the first 12 hours after birth. It is useful to establish a record-keeping system so that client compliance can be measured. For example, dates and times that procedures took place can be recorded with the initials of the individual responsible for the task.

Monitor progress

Outbreak investigations provide an educable moment for many cattle producers. This time may be right to convince herd managers of the value of an animal health and performance record-keeping system.[65,66] Records help validate that the corrective actions are working and a process control approach may catch problems before they become costly or harmful to calf health and well-being.[67]

SUMMARY

Diarrhea is a leading cause of sickness and death of beef and dairy calves in their first month of life. Field investigations of outbreaks of neonatal calf diarrhea should be conducted for the purposes of (1) reducing the losses associated with existing cases and (2) preventing new cases from occurring.

Outbreak investigations for any infectious or toxicant-induced disease involve an orderly process of characterizing the outbreak and finding solutions using epidemiologic concepts that include the following:

- Interviewing key individuals
- Verifying the clinical diagnosis and assure that treatments are appropriate

- Identifying the factors responsible for the outbreak using a rational diagnostic plan and qualitative or quantitative analytical methods
- Developing strategies to prevent new cases and future outbreaks by identifying corrective actions likely to have the most impact without excessive cost
- Communicating observations and recommendations with the key individuals, and using records to verify compliance and monitor progress.

REFERENCES

1. USDA. Part II: reference of 1997 beef cow-calf health and management practices. Fort Collins (CO): USDA, APHIS, VS, CEAH, National Animal Health Monitoring System; 1997.
2. Anderson DC, Kress DD, Bernardini MM, et al. The effect of scours on calf weaning weight. Prof Anim Sci 2003;19:399–403.
3. Swift BL, Nelms GE, Coles R. The effect of neonatal diarrhea on subsequent weight gains in beef calves. Vet Med Small Anim Clin 1976;71(9):1269–72.
4. Smith DR. Management of neonatal diarrhea in cow-calf herds. In: Anderson DE, Rings DM, editors. Current veterinary therapy food animal practice. 5th edition. St Louis (MO): Saunders Elsevier; 2009. p. 599–602.
5. Waldner CL, Campbell JR. Disease outbreak investigation in food animal practice. Vet Clin North Am Food Anim Pract 2006;22(1):75–101.
6. Hancock DD, Wikse SE. Investigation planning and data gathering. Vet Clin North Am Food Anim Pract 1988;4:1–15.
7. Lessard PR. The characterization of disease outbreaks. Vet Clin North Am Food Anim Pract 1988;4:17–32.
8. Mason GL, Madden DJ. Performing the field necropsy examination. Vet Clin North Am Food Anim Pract 2007;23(3):503–26, vi.
9. Acres SD, Laing CJ, Saunders JR, et al. Acute undifferentiated neonatal diarrhea in beef calves. I. Occurrence and distribution of infectious agents. Can J Comp Med 1975;39(2):116–32.
10. Acres SD, Saunders JR, Radostits OM. Acute undifferentiated neonatal diarrhea of beef calves: the prevalence of enterotoxigenic *E. coli*, reo-like (rota) virus and other enteropathogens in cow-calf herds. Can Vet J 1977;18(5):274–80.
11. Saif LJ, Smith KL. Enteric viral infections of calves and passive immunity. J Dairy Sci 1985;68(1):206–28.
12. Barrington GM, Gay JM, Evermann JF. Biosecurity for neonatal gastrointestinal diseases. Vet Clin North Am Food Anim Pract 2002;18(1):7–34.
13. Bulgin MS, Anderson BC, Ward AC, et al. Infectious agents associated with neonatal calf disease in southwestern Idaho and eastern Oregon. J Am Vet Med Assoc 1982;180(10):1222–6.
14. Mebus CA, Stair EL, Rhodes MB, et al. Neonatal calf diarrhea: propagation, attenuation, and characteristics of coronavirus-like agents. Am J Vet Res 1973;34:145–50.
15. Trotz-Williams LA, Jarvie BD, Martin SW, et al. Prevalence of *Cryptosporidium parvum* infection in southwestern Ontario and its association with diarrhea in neonatal dairy calves. Can Vet J 2005;46(4):349–51.
16. Athanassious R, Marsollais G, Assaf R, et al. Detection of bovine coronavirus and type A rotavirus in neonatal calf diarrhea and winter dysentery of cattle in Quebec: evaluation of three diagnostic methods. Can Vet J 1994;35:163–9.
17. Naciri M, Lefay MP, Mancassola R, et al. Role of Cryptosporidium parvum as a pathogen in neonatal diarrhoea complex in suckling and dairy calves in France. Vet Parasitol 1999;85(4):245–57.

18. Morin M, Lariviere S, Lallier R. Pathological and microbiological observations made on spontaneous cases of acute neonatal calf diarrhea. Can J Comp Med 1976;40(3):228–40.
19. Lucchelli A, Lance SA, Bartlett PB, et al. Prevalence of bovine group A rotavirus shedding among dairy calves in Ohio. Am J Vet Res 1992;53:169–74.
20. Crouch CF, Bielefeldt Ohman H, Watts TC, et al. Chronic shedding of bovine enteric coronavirus antigen-antibody complexes by clinically normal cows. J Gen Virol 1985;66:1489–500.
21. Collins JK, Riegel CA, Olson JD, et al. Shedding of enteric coronavirus in adult cattle. Am J Vet Res 1987;48:361–5.
22. Crouch CF, Acres SD. Prevalence of rotavirus and coronavirus antigens in the feces of normal cows. Can J Comp Med 1984;48:340–2.
23. McAllister TA, Olson ME, Fletch A, et al. Prevalence of Giardia and Cryptosporidium in beef cows in southern Ontario and in beef calves in southern British Columbia. Can Vet J 2005;46(1):47–55.
24. Watanabe Y, Yang CH, Ooi HK. Cryptosporidium infection in livestock and first identification of *Cryptosporidium parvum* genotype in cattle feces in Taiwan. Parasitol Res 2005;97(3):238–41.
25. Ralston BJ, McAllister TA, Olson ME. Prevalence and infection pattern of naturally acquired giardiasis and cryptosporidiosis in range beef calves and their dams. Vet Parasitol 2003;114(2):113–22.
26. Smith DR. Epidemiologic tools for biosecurity and biocontainment. Vet Clin North Am Food Anim Pract 2002;18(1):157–75.
27. McKenna SL, Dohoo IR. Using and interpreting diagnostic tests. Vet Clin North Am Food Anim Pract 2006;22(1):195–205.
28. Barrington GM, Parish SM. Bovine neonatal immunology. Vet Clin North Am Food Anim Pract 2001;17(3):463–76.
29. Besser TE, Gay CC. The importance of colostrum to the health of the neonatal calf. Vet Clin North Am Food Anim Pract 1994;10(1):107–17.
30. Besser TE, Gay CC, McGuire TC, et al. Passive immunity to bovine rotavirus infection associated with transfer of serum antibody into the intestinal lumen. J Virol 1988;62(7):2238–42.
31. Clement JC, King ME, Salman MD, et al. Use of epidemiologic principles to identify risk factors associated with the development of diarrhea in calves in five beef herds. J Am Vet Med Assoc 1995;207(10):1334–8.
32. Smith DR, Grotelueschen DM, Knott T, et al. Population dynamics of undifferentiated neonatal calf diarrhea among ranch beef calves. Bovine Practitioner 2008; 42(8):1–8.
33. El-Kanawati ZR, Tsunemitsu H, Smith DR, et al. Infection and cross-protection studies of winter dysentery and calf diarrhea bovine coronavirus strains in colostrum-deprived and gnotobiotic calves. Am J Vet Res 1996;57:48–53.
34. Heckert RA, Saif LJ, Mengel JP, et al. Mucosal and systemic antibody responses to bovine coronavirus structural proteins in experimentally challenge-exposed calves fed low or high amounts of colostral antibodies. Am J Vet Res 1991;52(5):700–8.
35. Saif LJ, Redman DR, Moorhead PD, et al. Experimentally induced coronavirus infections in calves: viral replication in the respiratory and intestinal tracts. Am J Vet Res 1986;47:1426–32.
36. Kapil S, Trent AM, Goyal SM. Excretion and persistence of bovine coronavirus in neonatal calves. Arch Virol 1990;115:127–32.
37. Uga S, Matsuo J, Kono E, et al. Prevalence of *Cryptosporidium parvum* infection and pattern of oocyst shedding in calves in Japan. Vet Parasitol 2000;94(1–2):27–32.

38. Nydam DV, Wade SE, Schaaf SL, et al. Number of *Cryptosporidium parvum* oocysts of *Giardia* spp. cysts by dairy calves after natural infection. Am J Vet Res 2001;62(10):1612–5.
39. O'Handley RM, Cockwill C, McAllister TA, et al. Duration of naturally acquired giardiasis and cryptosporidiosis in dairy calves and their association with diarrhea. J Am Vet Med Assoc 1999;214(3):391–6.
40. Murakami Y, Nishioka N, Watanabe T, et al. Prolonged excretion and failure of cross-protection between distinct serotypes of bovine rotavirus. Vet Microbiol 1986;12(1):7–14.
41. Schumann FJ, Townsend HG, Naylor JM. Risk factors for mortality from diarrhea in beef calves in Alberta. Can J Vet Res 1990;54(3):366–72.
42. Odde KG. Reducing neonatal calf losses through selection, nutrition and management. Agri-Practice 1996;17(3/4):12–5.
43. Odde KG. Survival of the neonatal calf. Vet Clin North Am Food Anim Pract 1988; 4:501–8.
44. Law J. Diseases of young calves. Special report on diseases of cattle. Washington, DC: United States Department of Agriculture, Bureau of Animal Industry; 1916. p. 245–61.
45. Van Es L. White scours. The principles of animal hygiene and preventive veterinary medicine. New York: John Wiley and Sons, Inc.; 1932. p. 504–13.
46. Atwill ER, Johnson EM, Pereira MG. Association of herd composition, stocking rate, and duration of calving season with fecal shedding of Cryptosporidium parvum oocysts in beef herds. J Am Vet Med Assoc 1999;215(12):1833–8.
47. Rothman KJ. Causes. Am J Epidemiol 1976;104:587–92.
48. Gay JM. Determining cause and effect in herds. Vet Clin North Am Food Anim Pract 2006;22(1):125–47.
49. Koch R. Die aetiologie der tuberkulose. Mitt Kaiser Gesundh 1884;2:1–88 [in German].
50. Hill AB. The environment and disease: association or causation? Proc R Soc Med 1965;58:295–300.
51. Susser M. What is a cause and how do we know one? A grammar for pragmatic epidemiology. Am J Epidemiol 1991;133:635–48.
52. Evans AS. Causation and disease: a chronological journey. Am J Epidemiol 1978; 108:249–58.
53. Shott S. Designing studies that answer questions. J Am Vet Med Assoc 2011; 238(1):55–8.
54. Slenning BD. Hood of the truck statistics for food animal practitioners. Vet Clin North Am Food Anim Pract 2006;22(1):149–70.
55. Dargatz DA, Garry FB, Traub-Dargatz JL. An introduction to biosecurity of cattle operations. Vet Clin North Am Food Anim Pract 2002;18(1):1–5.
56. Larson RL, Tyler JW, Schultz LG, et al. Management strategies to decrease calf death losses in beef herds. J Am Vet Med Assoc 2004;224(1):42–8.
57. Nocek JE, Braund DG, Warner RG. Influence of neonatal colostrum administration, immunoglobulin, and continued feeding of colostrum on calf gain, health, and serum protein. J Dairy Sci 1984;67(2):319–33.
58. Lu W, Duhamel GE, Benfield DA, et al. Serological and genotypic characterization of group A rotavirus reassortants from diarrheic calves born to dams vaccinated against rotavirus. Vet Microbiol 1994;42(2–3):159–70.
59. Sanders DE. Field management of neonatal diarrhea. Vet Clin North Am Food Anim Pract 1985;1(3):621–37.

60. Radostits OM, Acres SD. The control of acute undifferentiated diarrhea of newborn beef calves. Vet Clin North Am Large Anim Pract 1983;5(1):143–55.
61. Thomson JU. Implementing biosecurity in beef and dairy herds. Proc Am Assoc Bov Pract 1997;30:8–14.
62. Pence M, Robbe S, Thomson J. Reducing the incidence of neonatal calf diarrhea through evidence-based management. Compendium on Continuing Education for the Practicing Veterinarian 2001;23:S73–5.
63. Smith DR, Grotelueschen DM, Knott T, et al. Prevention of neonatal calf diarrhea with the Sandhills calving system. Proc Am Assoc Bov Pract 2004;37:166–8.
64. Sanderson MW. Designing and running clinical trials on farms. Vet Clin North Am Food Anim Pract 2006;22(1):103–23.
65. Rae DO. Assessing performance of cow-calf operations using epidemiology. Vet Clin North Am Food Anim Pract 2006;22(1):53–74.
66. Kelton DF. Epidemiology: a foundation for dairy production medicine. Vet Clin North Am Food Anim Pract 2006;22(1):21–33.
67. Reneau JK, Lukas J. Using statistical process control methods to improve herd performance. Vet Clin North Am Food Anim Pract 2006;22(1):171–93.

Gross Lesions of Alimentary Disease in Adult Cattle

Bradley L. Njaa, DVM, MVSc[a],*, Roger J. Panciera, DVM, PhD[a],
Edward G. Clark, DVM, MVSc[b], Catherine G. Lamm, DVM, MRCVS[c]

KEYWORDS

• Gross lesions • Alimentary disease • Cattle • Necropsy • Enteritis

KEY POINTS

- Gross lesions in the gastrointestinal tract must be incorporated with clinical and historical data to provide meaningful interpretations.
- Red bowel typifies congestion more commonly than hemorrhage or hemorrhagic enteritis.
- Enteritis usually includes, in addition to congestion or hemorrhage, edema, fibrin or feed material adherent to affected mucosa, mucosal erosion, ulcers or necrosis, serosal hemorrhage with adherent fibrin, and luminal contents with abnormal consistency and possibly a miasmic odor.

NECROPSY EXAMINATION

Gross examination of the gastrointestinal tract (GIT) of cattle is one of the most challenging parts of a necropsy. The GIT is one of the largest and heaviest organ systems of the animal. It is initially divided into the upper GIT (oral cavity, esophagus, forestomachs, abomasum) and the lower GIT (intestines, rectum, and anus). In healthy cattle, the forestomachs occupy more than half the abdominal cavity. The rumen (**Fig. 1**) alone has a capacity range of 102 to 148 L (which approximates to a similar weight in kilograms), whereas the abomasal volume ranges from 10 to 20 L.[1] The intestines occupy a much smaller space in the peritoneal cavity but have a length that is considerable, ranging from 33 to 63 m.[1] Thus, a thorough examination is physically demanding because of its size and requires a significant proportion of time to adequately examine its entirety.

In addition, the GIT is one of the few organ systems that normally contain a mixture of commensal and potentially pathogenic organisms. In health, there is continuous interaction between the host and microorgansims resulting in a perpetual steady state

[a] Department of Pathobiology, Center for Veterinary Health Sciences, Oklahoma State University, 250 McElroy Hall, Stillwater, OK 74074–2007, USA; [b] 71 Douglasview Road Southeast, Calgary, Alberta T2Z 2S8, Canada; [c] School of Veterinary Medicine, University of Glasgow, Bearsden, Glasgow, UK
* Corresponding author.
E-mail address: brad.njaa@okstate.edu

Vet Clin Food Anim 28 (2012) 483–513
http://dx.doi.org/10.1016/j.cvfa.2012.07.009
0749-0720/12/$ – see front matter © 2012 Elsevier Inc. All rights reserved.

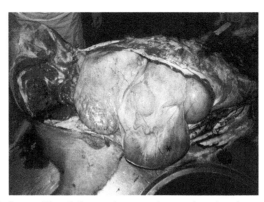

Fig. 1. Abdominal viscera. The abdomen is opened, exposing the viscera. The forestomachs occupy most of the abdominal space. Typically, the abomasum (*asterisk*) is a darker reddish purple compared with the forestomachs. (*Courtesy* Dr E.G. Clark, Western College of Veterinary Medicine, University of Saskatchewan, Saskatoon, SK.)

of controlled inflammation. Once the animal dies, these organisms continue to rapidly proliferate, are exothermic, and release destructive enzymes and gases that lead to rapid autolytic and putrefactive changes that can quickly obfuscate the superficial intestinal mucosa either obscuring lesions or creating pseudolesions. Timely examination of the GIT is essential for the best opportunity to contribute to the diagnostic process.

For ease of examination during necropsy, the gastrointestinal system is divided into three to four sections: the oral cavity and esophagus; the forestomachs and true stomach (abomasum); and the intestines, which can be divided into small and large intestines separately or examined as a continuum. Examination of the GIT begins with a thorough examination of the oral cavity, including the lips, gums, hard and soft palate, teeth, and tongue for erosions, ulceration, hemorrhage, and masses. Remember that many esophageal lesions tend to be in the distal one-third of the esophagus.

It is important to be thorough to detect subtle mucosal erosions or ulcers, find stray wire or lead particles in the reticulum, identify parts of toxic plants in all compartments, characterize the feed, or observe substances that are not miscible in water-based rumen contents. These changes can be easily overlooked or missed if this part of the necropsy is given a cursory glance or omitted all together. All four compartments must be thoroughly opened and their contents evacuated to better examine the mucosa.

Ideally, the small and large intestine should be stripped from its mesenteric attachments before or during removal from the peritoneal cavity allowing palpation for masses, recognition of any color variation, and localization of any areas of serosal inflammation or perforations. A good place to begin is where the ileum attaches to the cecum and begin stripping orally toward the duodenum. Identifying the ileum is also important because it is a common location for many intestinal diseases and ensures that Peyer's patches are located and collected. Resist the temptation to only "spot check" various segments of the intestine because subtle or regionally variable lesions could be easily missed.

While opening segments of intestine to assess contents, the mucosa can be more thoroughly evaluated. The often semifluid to pasty consistency of intestinal contents may obscure the mucosa beneath impairing its thorough examination. It is tempting to scrape this material off of the mucosa with the edge of the necropsy knife, but that damages the underlying epithelium if histopathology is desired. If that is the only means of assessment, then ensure that other segments with similar gross lesions are sampled for histopathology. Small amounts of water under low pressure or small amounts poured over the mucosa more gently clear the contents from the surface and allow more detailed examination. If a pathogen is suspected, representative sections of bowel should be collected for microbiologic testing before opening or flushing the segments. Ensure that segments of intestine collected for microbial testing are kept closed, using string to seal the ends of the segments. When submitting to the laboratory, it is imperative that segments of bowel are packaged separately from other fresh tissues.

The purpose of the gross necropsy examination of the GIT is to recognize the presence of lesions, thus requiring a basic understanding of its normal appearance and anatomy. This article highlights gross changes to the GIT of adult cattle that help place the disease process into broad categories. Although few gross lesions reach the zenith of pathognomonic, there are numerous lesions that when considered in aggregate with history (number of animals affected, environment, duration of signs, time of onset relative to management changes, previous management, and so forth) and clinical signs can help narrow the spectrum of causes, provide a basis for a strong presumptive diagnosis, and focus diagnostic test selection.

LESION CATEGORIZATION

There are numerous ways to codify gastrointestinal gross pathology. One of the most practical methods is to classify lesions using the following broad categories: color variation, mucosal surface integrity, size variation, and luminal content features. Each category is briefly introduced in general broad terms. For each functional and anatomic division, normal is defined followed by application of the method to each segment. The GIT is divided into the oropharynx, esophagus, forestomachs, abomasum, and intestines.

GENERAL CONSIDERATIONS
Color Changes

Red mucosa in the abomasum and intestines is often normal or uninterpretable as it relates to disease or inflammation but is commonly misdiagnosed as hemorrhage and inflammation (**Fig. 2**). Many dead cattle can have segments of quite red intestine, even with bloody contents, that histologically do not translate into hemorrhage or inflammation. Smudgy red to pink discoloration of gastrointestinal serosa is frequently encountered in adult cattle with prolonged postmortem intervals caused by lysis of red cells with leakage or imbibition of hemoglobin into the tissue interstitium. With time and proliferation of bacteria, imbibed hemoglobin can react with bacteria-derived hydrogen sulfide to produce iron-containing compounds that impart a dark green to black tissue discoloration, referred to as "pseudomelanosis."

Serosal surfaces of the forestomachs, abomasum, and intestines tend to be highly variable, ranging from pale tan to pink to medium purple, dependent largely on the postmortem interval. Never judge an animal as pale based solely on serosal surface pallor. Serosa may be helpful along with subcutaneous tissues in detecting and confirming icterus.

Mucosal Surface Integrity

In general, mucosal surfaces have a glistening sheen that is best mimicked by visual appearance of "semigloss" to "glossy" finish house paints. When mucous membranes have a texture that is analogous to "matte" or "eggshell" paint finishes, that is strongly suggestive of erosion or shallow ulcers. When the center of defects is brighter or

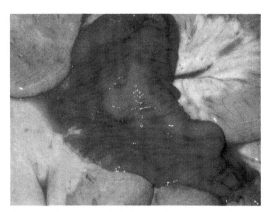

Fig. 2. Congested jejunum. The mucosa is intensely hyperemic, which can be normal. This is not considered enteritis because there is a lack of blotchy hemorrhage, the mucosa has a prominent, velvety sheen, and there is no evidence of fibrinous exudation. The serosal surfaces look normal. (*Courtesy* Dr B. Hoff, Animal Health Laboratory, University of Guelph, Guelph, ON.)

darker red compared with the surrounding glistening mucosa, that is strongly suggestive of ulceration. Adherent feed or fibrin to the mucosal surface is a strong indication of local necrosis and inflammation.

Size Variation

Variation in the size of segments of the GIT tends to be the result of changes in wall thickness and luminal diameter. In general, increases in mural thickness can be caused by physiologic hypertrophy to the tunica muscularis or mucosal epithelium or by expansion of selected lamina or all layers of the wall because of accumulation of excess fluid or gas, infiltration by inflammatory cells, neoplasia, or a combination. Mural thickness may be decreased in cases where the luminal diameter is greatly expanded causing mural stretching or in cases where there is mural necrosis.

Excess fluid collected in tissues can be an antemortem physiologic response to hypoproteinemia leading to edema; it can result from localized or systemic inflammation, or possibly a response to excessive intravenous administration of fluid. Postmortem fluid accumulation can occur if the postmortem interval to necropsy is prolonged or if the carcass remains in an environment with high ambient temperatures and relative humidity. Similarly, excessive expansion by gas may be caused by antemortem proliferation of gas-producing bacteria, complications related to previous surgery, or disease. More commonly, excess gas accumulation in a carcass occurs postmortem related to proliferation of gas-producing anaerobic bacteria, such as *Clostridium* spp.

Luminal diameter is dependent on the muscular and neural integrity of the viscus wall, the transit time of the luminal contents, and the balance between absorption and secretion in the various segments of the GIT. Any alteration to one or more of these components can dramatically affect the size of the GIT, especially the intestines. For example, a focal intestinal obstruction can lead to proximal accumulation of fluid and resultant distention along with collapse or narrowing of the distal bowel (**Fig. 3**).

Luminal Content Features

Luminal contents are normally variable depending on the segment being examined in terms of odor, consistency, and color. Factors that contribute to this include type of diet (pasture vs dry lot vs feedlot rations); amount and type of water consumption;

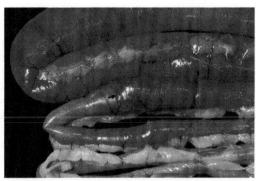

Fig. 3. Focal small intestinal obstruction. An intraluminal obstruction (*arrow*) is present, resulting in a markedly dilated and congested proximal bowel and mostly empty distal bowel. (*Courtesy* Dr B.L. Njaa, Center for Veterinary Health Sciences, Oklahoma State University, Stillwater, OK.)

and concurrent stressors, such as animal density, environmental stressors, and disease. Ruminal contents tend to have a sweet aromatic scent when cattle are on pasture or fed silage but become more sour and acidic in the face of high-grain diets or in cases of acidosis. Intestinal contents tend to move from coarse to liquid to pasty to semisolid when moving from oral to anal. Deviation from this often correlates with various disease states. Finally, color is extremely variable throughout the bowel and only in few circumstances is it diagnostically useful.

PATHOLOGY OF SPECIFIC ANATOMIC LOCATIONS WITHIN THE GIT
Oropharynx

Oropharyngeal mucosa tends to be highly variable in terms of melanin pigmentation depending on the breed and color variations within particular breeds. Dorsally, the dental pad is a thickened, often fissured area that apposes the lower incisor teeth. Teeth tend to have white enamel with darker green to brown to black staining of the opposing surface of upper and lower arcades.

Oral mucosa typically has a bright, slightly moist sheen. The hard palate has transverse ridges from which caudally project papillae that help guide food in an aboral direction. The soft palate is continuous with the hard palate and tends to have a smooth surface. The cheek mucosa has long, broad, aborally directed papillae that are sharply pointed in health (**Fig. 4**).

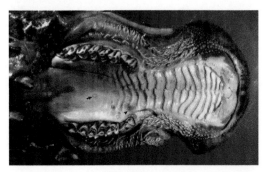

Fig. 4. Bovine papular stomatitis involving the oropharynx. Numerous circular (*arrow*) lesions are scattered throughout the surface of the hard and soft palate. Several of the lesions are less circular and have a more proliferative superficial exudation (*arrowhead*). (*Courtesy* College of Veterinary Medicine, Cornell University, Ithaca, NY.)

Tongues are their principle organ of prehension in cattle. Overlying the dorsal surface of the tongue are small, fine, sharp papillae, many of which play a sensory role. Approximately three-fifths caudal to the rostral tip is the lingual fossa demarcating the rostral edge of a large dorsal prominence called the *torus linguae*.[2]

Brown to blackened teeth with hypoplastic enamel is likely caused by chronic fluorosis (**Fig. 5**). Alternatively, hypoplastic or dysplastic enamel can be the result of *in utero* bovine viral diarrhea virus (BVDV) infections (**Fig. 6**). Oropharyngeal mucous membranes can become pale because of anemia or severe blood loss. Alternatively, they can become cyanotic because of cardiovascular compromise and collapse. When a cow is exposed to high nitrate–containing plants (frost-damaged cereal crops, *Brassicaceae* spp, and *Sorghum* spp) or fertilizers, the nitrate is converted to nitrite and when it is absorbed converts hemoglobin to methemoglobin, imparting a light brown or "muddy" tincture to blood and tissues (**Fig. 7**).

Localized and systemic diseases with inherent epitheliotropism may first be visualized when examining the oropharynx but are rarely limited to this location. Shallow erosions tend to be slightly different from the surrounding tissue because of pigmentation changes and loss of the typical sheen (**Fig. 8**). Similar lesions may be seen in the lingual mucosa (**Fig. 9**). Causes frequently associated with this lesion include BVDV, bluetongue virus (BTV), herpes viruses that cause malignant catarrhal fever (MCF), rinderpest, and rupture of epithelial vesicles.

Vesicular disease is a category of disease that typically involves a certain degree of alarm and investigation and confirmatory testing by federal veterinarians. In North America, these most often are categorized as foreign animal diseases or transboundary animal diseases. Commonly, intact vesicles or erosions, the result of ruptured vesicles, are the first sign of concern, initially observed on the muzzle and in the oral cavity. Ruptured vesicles and erosions when secondarily infected, can become deep, inflamed, painful, mucosal ulcers. Possible causes include foot-and-mouth disease, vesicular stomatitis, chronic BVD, BTV, and MCF (**Fig. 10**).[3] Other causes that tend to lead to severe erosion or ulceration include blister beetle (cantharidin) toxicosis; traumatic injury secondary to coarse feeds or caustic chemicals; and uremia. In extreme cases, plant awns or hair may embed themselves in the ulcerated lingual mucosa, especially in the lingual fossa, giving the appearance of lingual "hair" (**Fig. 11**).

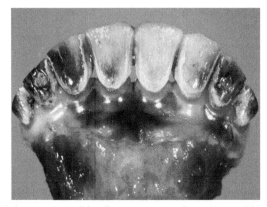

Fig. 5. Periodontal disease caused by fluorosis. Enamel erosion and hypoplasia and black discoloration are caused by excess fluoride ingestion. The white material on the surface of the teeth is what remains of the enamel. (*Courtesy* College of Veterinary Medicine, Cornell University, Ithaca, NY.)

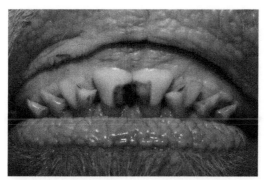

Fig. 6. Periodontal enamel defect caused by BVDV. This bilaterally symmetric enamel defect in deciduous incisor teeth is cause by a previous *in utero* infection with BVDV. (*Courtesy* Dr E.G. Clark, Western College of Veterinary Medicine, University of Saskatchewan, Saskatoon, SK.)

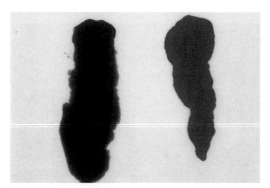

Fig. 7. Methemoglobinemia. The blood on the left is muddy, red brown, collected from an animal exposed to excess nitrates. The blood on the right is from a normal animal. (*Courtesy* Dr R.J. Panciera, Center for Veterinary Health Sciences, Oklahoma State University, Stillwater, OK.)

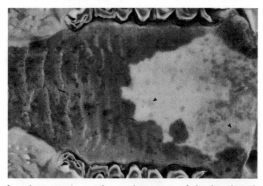

Fig. 8. Hard and soft palate erosions. The oral mucosa of the hard and soft palate is multi-focally eroded with areas (*arrowheads*) that lack the normal glistening sheen and are typically darker than the surrounding unaffected mucosa. BVDV was confirmed as the cause in this case based on enzyme-linked immunosorbent immunoassay and immunohistochemistry techniques. (*Courtesy* Dr B.L. Njaa, Center for Veterinary Health Sciences, Oklahoma State University, Stillwater, OK.)

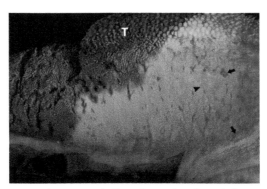

Fig. 9. Lingual erosions. There are shallow (*arrowhead*) and deeper erosions (*arrows*) affecting the mucosal surface of the tongue. The lingual papillae covering the surface of the torus linguae (T) are blunted. This is the tongue from the same animal in **Fig. 8** that was confirmed positive for BVDV. (*Courtesy* Dr B.L. Njaa, Center for Veterinary Health Sciences, Oklahoma State University, Stillwater, OK.)

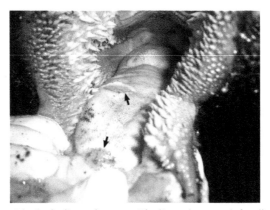

Fig. 10. Ruptured vesicles in the lingual mucosa. The lingual mucosa is focally ulcerated (*arrows*) in areas where vesicles have ruptured. This animal was a confirmed case of foot-and-mouth disease during an outbreak in Bolivia in 2007. (*Courtesy* Dr C. Orozco, USDA, APHIS, Bolivia.)

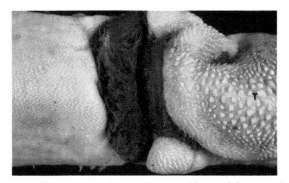

Fig. 11. Necroulcerative lingual gingivitis. At the rostral base of the *torus linguae* (T), in the lingual fossa is an area of dark red ulcerative inflammation within which are embedded grass awns mixed with other feed material. (*Courtesy* Dr E.G. Clark, Western College of Veterinary Medicine, University of Saskatchewan, Saskatoon, SK.)

Bovine viral diarrhea virus

- Erosive lesions in the alimentary mucosa are strongly suggestive of BVDV infections, whereas ulcerative lesions have a much broader spectrum of potential etiologies[13,19,20]

- BVDV is a pancytotropic virus that can replicate in nearly every cell type, thus most body systems are susceptible to infection

- In utero infection with BVD can result in persistently infected cattle

- Persistently infected cattle are key to maintaining BVDV in a bovine population

- BVDV infections may manifest as

  ○ Alimentary disease

  ○ Reproductive disease

  ○ Respiratory disease

  ○ Immunocompromized state with increased susceptibility to other infectious agents

  ○ Thrombocytopenic disease

- Diagnosis

  ○ Sample selection: whole blood, serum, milk, lymphoid tissue, gastrointestinal tissue, skin

  ○ Broad selection of tissues for microscopic examination

  ○ Test methodologies: virus isolation, fluorescent antibody testing, immunohistochemistry, enzyme-linked immunosorbent assay, reverse-transcriptase polymerase chain reaction

For more information on diagnostic testing rationale, please refer to reference.[20]

Two of the more commonly referred to ailments of the oropharynx that lead to swelling and variation in size are "lumpy jaw" and "wooden tongue." The former is also referred to as "actinomycosis," denoting a severe osteomyelitis that results from *Actinomyces bovis* penetration through the oropharyngeal mucosa with subsequent penetration of the periosteum of the mandible and eventual mandibular osteomyelitis.[4] This results in a severely disfiguring disease (**Fig. 12**). Wooden tongue, also called "actinobacillosis," is a lingual infection by *Actinobacillus lignieresii*. The tongue becomes markedly enlarged and painful and may develop ulceration because of its obstructive size and susceptibility to trauma (**Fig. 13**).[5]

Animals repeatedly exposed to bracken fern forage run the risk of developing squamous cell carcinoma of the upper GIT (**Fig. 14**).[6] Rarely, other neoplasms may affect the oropharynx leading to cachexia either through obstruction or because of impaired ability to masticate food.

Esophagus

Once opened and laid flat, the esophageal mucosa tends to be normally quite pale, with a smooth texture, lacking surface folds. The underlying submucosa is normally loosely attached to the overlying mucosa allowing for a moderate amount of laxity when the mucosa is torqued relative to the muscle layer.

At the level of the thoracic inlet is where a clearly demarcated line of congestion abruptly ends in pallor forming what is most commonly referred to as a "bloat line" (**Fig. 15**). This lesion occurs in cattle that develop markedly increased intra-abdominal pressure as ruminal pressure increases because of excess uneructated gas accumulation. This increased abdominal pressure compresses the thorax and blanches the intrathoracic portion of the esophagus, whereas the esophagus cranial

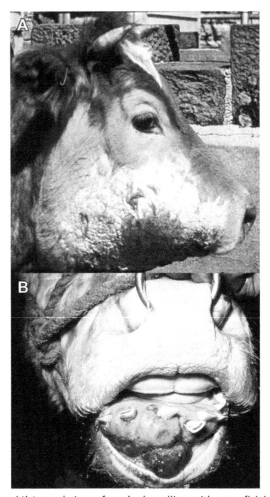

Fig. 12. Lumpy jaw. (*A*) Lateral view of marked swelling with superficial cutaneous ulceration and exudation. Most of the swelling is caused by boney proliferation associated with osteomyelitis. Most commonly, *Actinomyces bovis* is cultured from these lesions. (*B*) Rostral view of severe mandibular osteomyelitis with marked distortion of the mandibular incisors. (*Courtesy* Dr E.G. Clark, Western College of Veterinary Medicine, University of Saskatchewan, Saskatoon, SK.)

to the thoracic inlet tends to be markedly congested.[7] Any reason to prevent eructation of gas can lead to the formation of a bloat line.

Serpentine, pale white to orange red spirurid parasites are commonly found burrowed in the epithelium of the esophagus, and occasionally the lingual mucosa. This is the typical presentation of *Gongylonema pulchrum* infestations.[8] When present in the ruminal submucosa, they are *Gongylonema verrucosum*.[9] They are clinically inconsequential (**Fig. 16**).

Papules that form in the esophageal mucosa and oral mucosa (see **Fig. 4**) are very common in younger cattle, most often the result of bovine papular stomatitis virus, a member of the genus *Parapoxvirus*. Transmission probably occurs through direct contact and stress or immunosuppression may precipitate disease.[10] These lesions

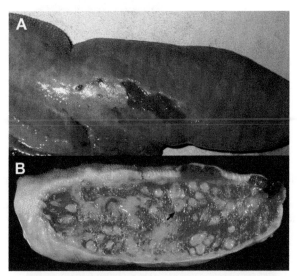

Fig. 13. Actinobacillosis or "wooden" tongue. (*A*) The tongue is markedly enlarge with several areas of chronic ulceration along its lateral edge. (*B*) Cross section through a case of wooden tongue with numerous pyogranulomas (*arrow*) scattered throughout the tongue. This is typically caused by *Actinobacillus lignieresii.* ([A] *Courtesy* Dr R.J. Panciera, Center for Veterinary Health Sciences, Oklahoma State University, Stillwater, OK; [B] *Courtesy* Dr E.G. Clark, Western College of Veterinary Medicine, University of Saskatchewan, Saskatoon, SK.)

are variable in size, typically very round to oval, and can be subtle raised foci or very prominent papules with raised rims and eroded centers and have adherent fibrin and feed material (**Fig. 17**). Erosions can affect the esophagus with causes similar to those described for the oropharynx (BVD, MCF, BTV) (**Fig. 18**). Deeper ulcerated lesions may be the result of secondarily infected BVD erosions, mucosal disease, MCF, infectious bovine rhinotracheitis, ruptured vesicles, or mucosal trauma (**Fig. 19**).[3]

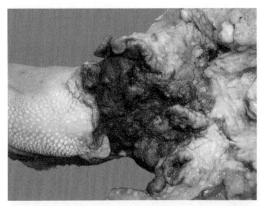

Fig. 14. Lingual and pharyngeal squamous cell carcinoma. A large area of ulceration is present at the base of the tongue. This was associated with chronic ingestion of bracken fern. (*From* Masuda EK, Kommers GD, Martins TB, et al. Morphologic factors as indicators of malignancy of squamous cell carcinomas in cattle exposed naturally to bracken fern (*Pteridium aquilium*). J Comp Pathol 2011;144:48–54; with permission.)

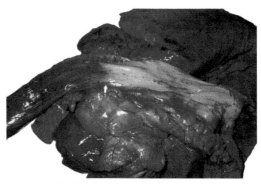

Fig. 15. Bloat line. Cranial to the level of the thoracic inlet (*arrow*), the esophagus is markedly congested, whereas caudal to this the esophagus is pale. This is an indication that elevated intraruminal pressure could not be alleviated resulting in severe vascular compromise and formation of a "bloat line." (*Courtesy* Dr R.J. Panciera, Center for Veterinary Health Sciences, Oklahoma State University, Stillwater, OK.)

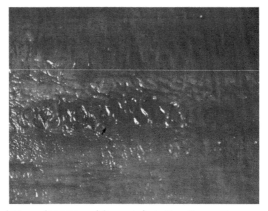

Fig. 16. Esophageal *Gongylonema pulchrum* infestation. Serpentine mucosal or submucosal parasites in the esophagus (*arrow*) are typical of *G pulchrum* infestation. When found in the rumen, they are *Gongylonema verrucosum*. (*Courtesy* Dr M. Czajkowski, College of Veterinary Medicine, Cornell University, Ithaca, NY.)

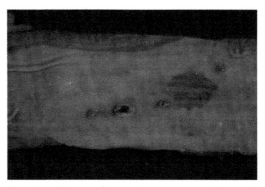

Fig. 17. Bovine papular stomatitis, esophagus. Numerous round to oval papules are present. The largest one is centrally ulcerated. Bovine papular stomatitis virus, often affecting cattle that may have impaired immunity, causes these lesions. (*Courtesy* Dr B.L. Njaa, Center for Veterinary Health Sciences, Oklahoma State University, Stillwater, OK.)

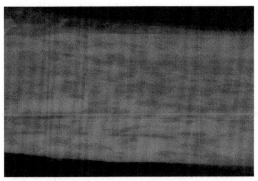

Fig. 18. Multifocal linear esophageal erosions. Numerous mucosal erosions are scattered throughout this esophagus. With lesions this numerous and shallow, BVD must be strongly considered. This animal was confirmed positive for BVDV. (*Courtesy* Dr B.L. Njaa, Center for Veterinary Health Sciences, Oklahoma State University, Stillwater, OK.)

Mucosal injury to the esophagus tends to heal by fibrosis and scarring resulting in luminal narrowing and stricture formation near the site of injury (**Fig. 20**). Injury may be caused by luminal foreign bodies that become lodged or any of the other infectious causes. Proximal to the stricture, the esophagus may become dilated

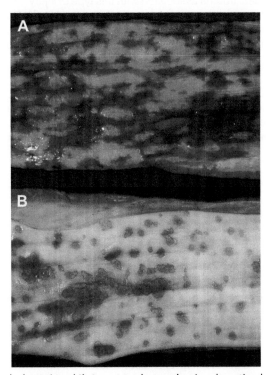

Fig. 19. Esophageal ulceration. (*A*) An acute, hemorrhagic, ulcerative lesion affecting the esophageal mucosa. (*B*) A subacute ulcerative esophagitis with superficial crusting. ([*A*] *Courtesy* Indiana Animal Disease Diagnostic Laboratory, Purdue University, West Lafayette, IN; [*B*] *Courtesy* Dr E.G. Clark, Western College of Veterinary Medicine, University of Saskatchewan, Saskatoon, SK.)

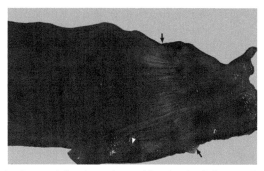

Fig. 20. Esophageal stricture. A focal esophageal foreign body has resulted in areas of ulceration (*white arrowhead*) and a circumferential area of pallor and constriction (*arrows*). (*Courtesy* Dr R.J. Panciera, Center for Veterinary Health Sciences, Oklahoma State University, Stillwater, OK.)

because of slowed or impaired passage of ingesta into the forestomachs. Periesophageal fasciitis that can result from "balling gun" injuries can cause esophageal luminal narrowing (**Fig. 21**). Traumatic injury from boluses forcibly ejected into the surrounding periesophageal tissue results in localized tissue damage, edema, and inflammation. In addition, pharyngeal trauma associated with this type of injury can result in acquired megaesophagus presumably caused by vagal nerve injury.[11] Rarely, intraluminal, mural, or periesophageal neoplasia can result in obstruction, luminal narrowing or dilation, dependent on either direct or indirect effects on esophageal function (**Fig. 22**).

Forestomachs

Forestomachs represent large, mucosal-lined, fluid-filled, and microbe-laden fermentation vats that are necessary for ruminants to convert the complex carbohydrates of plants into absorbable fatty acids. During the course of the digestion and fermentation

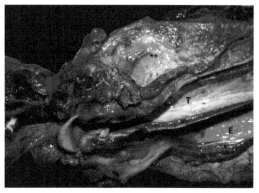

Fig. 21. Pharyngeal and periesophageal cellulitis or fasciitis. Both the trachea (T) and esophagus (E) have been displaced by a regional area of necrosis and inflammation (**). Any type of forceful injury to the pharynx can result in perforation, edema, necrosis, and inflammation. In this case, it was caused by improperly administered medicinal boluses by a mechanical dispensing device (ie, balling gun). (*Courtesy* Dr E.G. Clark, Western College of Veterinary Medicine, University of Saskatchewan, Saskatoon, SK.)

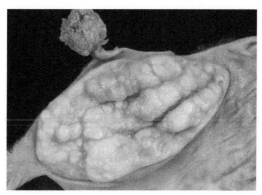

Fig. 22. Esophageal papillomatosis. A regional area of mucosal proliferation is present in the distal esophagus and a focal, pedunculated mass. Both are papillomas. (*Courtesy* Dr B.L. Njaa, Center for Veterinary Health Sciences, Oklahoma State University, Stillwater, OK.)

process, gases are produced along with thermal energy. Continued health of ruminants requires coordinated release of the fermentation gases produced and maintenance of rumen flora health. Alterations of this host-environment-microorganism homeostasis are what lead to lesions and disease.

The Reticulum

The reticulum or "honeycomb" is the most cranial, small, relative to the other forestomachs, sac comprising a mucosal web of interconnected, irregularly square, pentagonal or hexagonal, cells that are further divided into even smaller divisions.[12] Coarse, large, and heavy materials or objects tend to collect in the reticulum. Sharp objects indiscriminately ingested can accumulate in the reticulum resulting in an increased risk of mural penetration with consequences ranging from focal abscessation to peritonitis to diaphragmatic and pericardial perforation leading to a condition known as "traumatic reticulopericarditis" (**Fig. 23**). Ingestion of heavy material, such as lead, tends to collect in the mucosal-lined, ridged cells making this an important forestomach compartment to thoroughly examine (**Fig. 24**). Mucosal changes previously discussed can result in similar changes in the reticulum but are often missed because they are typically too subtle or the diagnosis is made based on lesions in other portions of the GIT (**Fig. 25**).

Rumen and Omasum

Forestomach mucosae tend to be greenish black because of staining by chlorophyll-containing feed. This staining tends to be relatively uniform throughout these compartments with the exception of the broad rumen pillars, which often are pale, lack papillae, and tend to have a thickened squamous mucosa. When the stained superficial layers of stratified squamous epithelium become blotchy, it is often an indication of disease processes that cause superficial erosions, such as BVD, MCF, or chemical rumenitis (**Fig. 26**). Similar blotchiness of the omasal mucosa is also typically seen. Any type of hemorrhagic diathesis can result in mural hemorrhages to any tissue or organ system. One cause to keep in mind is the acute hemorrhagic and thrombocytopenic form of acute BVD (**Fig. 27**).[13]

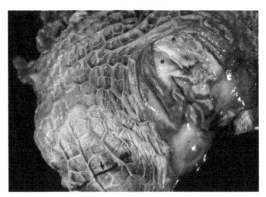

Fig. 23. Reticuloperitonitis. The reticulum is firmly adherent to the diaphragm with localized area of peritonitis (*asterisk*). A nail is embedded in the wall of the reticulum (*arrow*). It is most likely that this nail or another sharp, slender piece of metal penetrated through the wall of the reticulum to cause a localized peritonitis. If this inflammation tracks to the pericardial sac, it is called traumatic reticulopericarditis. (*Courtesy* Dr B.L. Njaa, Center for Veterinary Health Sciences, Oklahoma State University, Stillwater, OK.)

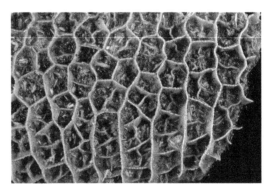

Fig. 24. Lead intoxication. Variably sized, sliver-gray, metallic particles are present within the mucosal compartments of the reticulum. These represent lead shavings obtained from a source of lead in a field, such as used batteries. (*Courtesy* Dr B.L. Njaa, Center for Veterinary Health Sciences, Oklahoma State University, Stillwater, OK.)

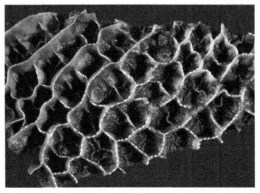

Fig. 25. Bovine papular stomatitis, reticulum. (*Courtesy* Dr R.J. Panciera, Center for Veterinary Health Sciences, Oklahoma State University, Stillwater, OK.)

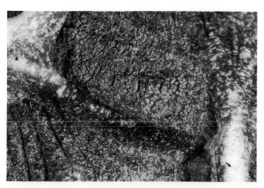

Fig. 26. Mucosal erosion, rumen. Early indication of shallow mucosal erosions is the loss of the normal greenish black coloration of the mucosa (*arrowhead*). Closer inspection reveals numerous shallow erosions in the mucosa (*arrow*). This case was confirmed BVDV positive. (*Courtesy* Dr B.L. Njaa, Center for Veterinary Health Sciences, Oklahoma State University, Stillwater, OK.)

Ulceration and mural necrosis can be seen in cases of necrobacillosis and mycotic infections. Both conditions are typically secondary invasion of the forestomach mucosa by *Fusobacterium necrophurm* or fungal organisms after primary traumatic or chemically (acidosis) induced mucosal injury (**Fig. 28**). Necrobacillosis invades through the mucosa into the wall but rarely penetrates to the serosal surfaces (**Fig. 29**). However, mycotic infections can either be superficial mucosal proliferation caused by infections with *Candida albicans* (**Fig. 30**) or deep and transmural involving the ruminal serosa because of the propensity of many fungi (ie, *Aspergillus* spp, *Mucor* spp, *Absidia* spp, *Rhizoporus* spp) to not only proliferate in squamous epithelium but also in the walls of blood vessels causing deep inflammation and infarction (**Fig. 31**).[11]

Ruminal mucosa varies from lacking papilla along the pillars to being densely covered by rumen papilla that range in length and size depending on the predominant feed-associated volatile fatty acids produced in the rumen fluid. Physiologic thickening and lengthening of the ruminal villi tends to occur with feeds that result in higher

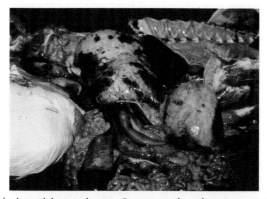

Fig. 27. Multifocal visceral hemorrhages. Forestomachs, abomasum, and intestines have mural hemorrhages. In this particular case, the cause was the thrombocytopenic form of BVD. (*Courtesy* Dr E.G. Clark, Western College of Veterinary Medicine, University of Saskatchewan, Saskatoon, SK.)

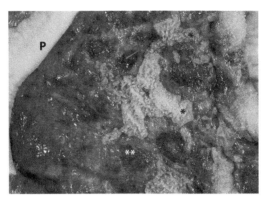

Fig. 28. Rumenitis. Arborizing islands of adherent mucosa cover small portions of the underlying submucosa (*asterisk*). The edges of these attached portions of epithelium are thickened and lack rumen papillae. These areas represent areas of rumenitis and epithelial injury. The remaining portions that lack epithelium represent normal postmortem sloughing of mucosa (**). P, rumen pillar. (*Courtesy* Dr E.G. Clark, Western College of Veterinary Medicine, University of Saskatchewan, Saskatoon, SK.)

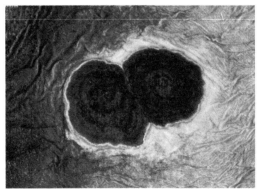

Fig. 29. Necrobacillosis. This focal area of necrosis is surrounded by a red rim of congestion. This represents a local response to proliferation of *Fusobacterium necrophorum*. (*Courtesy* Dr R.J. Panciera, Center for Veterinary Health Sciences, Oklahoma State University, Stillwater, OK.)

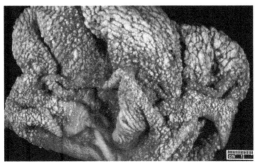

Fig. 30. Mucosal hyperplasia caused by superficial mycotic rumentitis, from *Candida albicans* proliferation. (*Courtesy* Indiana Animal Disease Diagnostic Laboratory, Purdue University, West Lafayette, IN.)

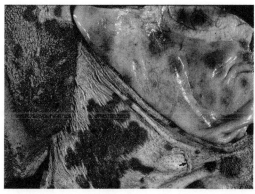

Fig. 31. Mycotic rumenitis. There are multifocal to coalescing areas of transmural hemorrhage affecting the rumen. These represent areas of fungal proliferation, on the surface squamous epithelium and in the walls of blood vessels. In this case, an initial ruminal acidosis caused by excess grain consumption caused significant mucosal injury allowing invasion and proliferation of fungi (ie, *Mucor* spp, or *Aspergillus* spp). In unaffected portions of the mucosa, the mucosal epithelium is lifting off in sheets (*arrow*). (*Courtesy* Dr R.J. Panciera, Center for Veterinary Health Sciences, Oklahoma State University, Stillwater, OK.)

levels of propionate and butyrate. Conversely, as the percent of dietary roughage increases, production of propionic and butyric acid decreases while ruminal acetic acid levels tend to increase, and ruminal mucosal papillar hypertrophy and hyperplasia does not occur.[11]

During necropsy examination of a normal adult bovid, the oral and esophageal mucosa remain firmly and tenaciously attached to the underlying submucosa, whereas the forestomach mucosa tends to normally lift off and away from the under-lying, typically reddened submucosa within a few hours of death (**Fig. 32**).[3] Conversely, easily sloughed oral and esophageal mucosa and firmly adherent forest-omach mucosa are indications of disease.

Parasitism of the ruminal mucosa can be challenging to observe and confirm without close inspection. Adult flukes that affect forestomachs of cattle from numerous genera are commonly grouped as paramphistome infections (**Fig. 33**). Adult

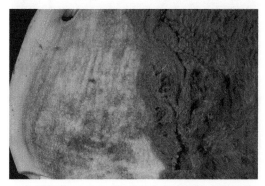

Fig. 32. Rumen mucosal epithelium normally sloughs easily from the submucosa several hours after death. If the rumen mucosal epithelium is firmly adherent, suspect a previous rumenitis (see **Fig. 28**). (*Courtesy* Dr B.L. Njaa, Center for Veterinary Health Sciences, Oklahoma State University, Stillwater, OK.)

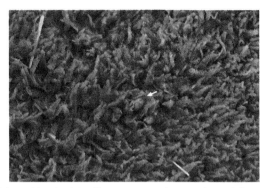

Fig. 33. Rumen flukes. Attached to the rumen surface and partially camouflaged by the rumen papillae are three rumen flukes (*arrow*). In this case, these are presumptively *Paramphistomum* spp. (*Courtesy* Mr. Richard Irvine and Dr C.G. Lamm, School of Veterinary Medicine, University of Glasgow, Glasgow, Scotland.)

parasites are red, pear-shaped, and tend to easily blend in with the rumen papillae but are typically incidental gross findings.[9]

Long, keratinized, papillary mucosal projections as the omasum opens into the reticulum and gastric groove are normal and referred to as unguiculliform papillae (**Fig. 34**).[14] However, proliferative lesions affecting the forestomachs can include papular stomatitis lesions (**Fig. 35**) and neoplasms, such as mural lymphoma, or mucosal epithelial neoplasms, such as fibropapillomas (**Fig. 36**).

Abomasum

Representing the true stomach of ruminants, this viscus is located caudal, ventral, and to the right of the rumen. It is typically slightly more purple than the forestomachs on its serosal surface and typically has a mucosa that is more red to reddish purple. The mucosal surface has much more of a wet, glistening sheen, lining a series of rugal folds.

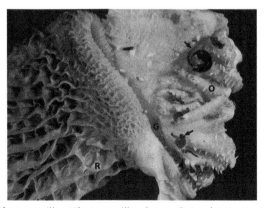

Fig. 34. Unguiculliform papillae. These papillae (*arrows*) may become quite prominent and gnarly near the reticular groove (G) along the junction of omasum (O) and reticulum (R) but are normal. (*Courtesy* Dr B.L. Njaa, Center for Veterinary Health Sciences, Oklahoma State University, Stillwater, OK.)

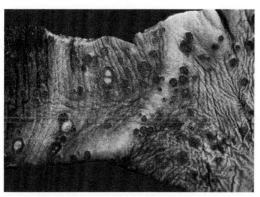

Fig. 35. Bovine papular stomatitis, rumen. (*Courtesy* Dr R.J. Panciera, Center for Veterinary Health Sciences, Oklahoma State University, Stillwater, OK.)

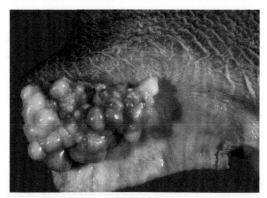

Fig. 36. Rumen papilloma. This focally proliferative, papillary growth is typical of a rumen papilloma. (*Courtesy* Dr R.J. Panciera, Center for Veterinary Health Sciences, Oklahoma State University, Stillwater, OK.)

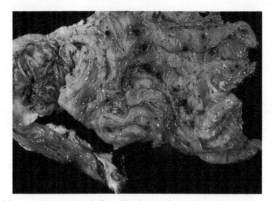

Fig. 37. Abomasal hemorrhage. Multifocally throughout the abomasal mucosa are variably sized dark red areas of hemorrhage. Any type of bleeding diathesis can result in this lesion. This particular example was a case of thrombocytopenic BVD. (*Courtesy* Dr E.G. Clark, Western College of Veterinary Medicine, University of Saskatchewan, Saskatoon, SK.)

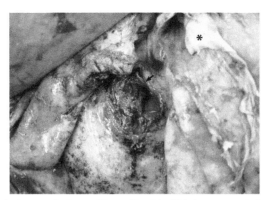

Fig. 38. Perforated abomasal ulcer with peritonitis. This is a serosal view of a perforated abomasal ulcer (*arrow*) that has resulted in a severe fibrinous peritonitis (*asterisk*). This is more commonly seen in young calves but less frequently can affect adult cattle. (*Courtesy* Dr B.L. Njaa, Center for Veterinary Health Sciences, Oklahoma State University, Stillwater, OK.)

Red, multifocal to confluent areas of hemorrhage in the abomasal mucosa are most often an indication of an ulcerative or infarction process (**Fig. 37**). Causes for such changes include various hemorrhagic diatheses including toxins (arsenic); corticosteroids (exogenous and endogenous); and infectious diseases (acute, thrombocytopenic, hemorrhagic BVD) (see **Fig. 27**). Perforating abomasal ulcers tend to affect young cattle. Less commonly, older animals may develop ulcerative lesions that eventually perforate and cause severe peritonitis (**Fig. 38**).

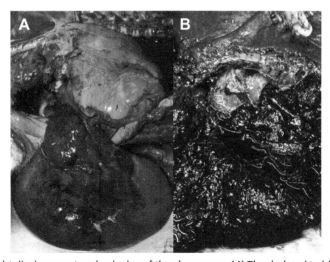

Fig. 39. Right displacement and volvulus of the abomasum. (*A*) The dark red to black viscus is the abomasum. Displacement and volvulus has resulted in severe vascular compromise and tissue death. (*B*) The mucosal surface of a similarly affected abomasum is extremely dark red and edematous caused by severe congestion and hemorrhage and necrosis. ([A] *Courtesy* Dr E.G. Clark, Western College of Veterinary Medicine, University of Saskatchewan, Saskatoon, SK; [B] *Courtesy* Dr B.L. Njaa, Center for Veterinary Health Sciences, Oklahoma State University, Stillwater, OK.)

Abomasal displacement and volvulus is a common condition affecting dairy cattle usually around the time of parturition. With the highest incidence in intensively managed herds, the abomasum typically displaces ventrally and to the left of the rumen. Less commonly, the abomasum displaces to the right increasing the chance for abomasal volvulus. The omasum is often involved in abomasal torsions. When severe, blood vessels in the neck of the omasum become obstructed resulting in not only organ distention but also severe congestion and hemorrhage (**Fig. 39**).[15]

Focal to diffuse mucosal thickening of abomasal rugal folds is characteristic of parasitism (**Fig. 40**). The lesion is a combination of mucous metaplasia and hyperplasia with associated chronic inflammation. The causes for this lesion include either *Ostertagia* spp or *Trichostrongylus axei*.[11]

The most common neoplasm that affects cattle is lymphoma. The abomasal wall is a predilection site (**Fig. 41**). Infiltration may be diffuse imparting a pale tan tincture to the entire affected area or multifocal, nodular infiltration of neoplastic lymphocytes. Other common sites for infiltration by neoplastic lymphocytes include forestomachs, heart, lymphoid organs, liver, reproductive tract, and spinal canal.[16]

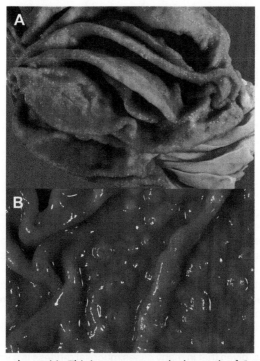

Fig. 40. Proliferative abomasitis. This is most commonly the result of *Ostertagia* spp infestation and associated inflammation. (*A*) Marked proliferation of all abomasal rugae. (*B*) Higher magnification of another example with focal areas of inflammation. ([*A*] *Courtesy* Dr R.J. Panciera, Center for Veterinary Health Sciences, Oklahoma State University, Stillwater, OK; [*B*] *Courtesy* Dr B.J. Johnson, California Animal Health and Food Safety Laboratory, University of California, Davis, CA.)

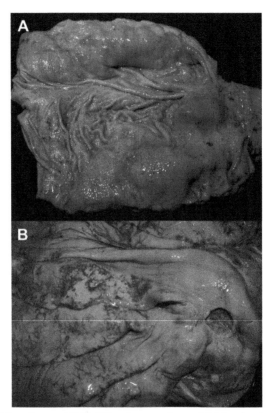

Fig. 41. Abomasal lymphoma. (*A*) Multifocal areas of mural thickening is one manifestation of abomasal lymphoma. (*B*) Most rugal folds in this abomasum are discolored pale tan and diffusely thickened because of infiltration by neoplastic lymphocytes. ([*A*] *Courtesy* Dr A.W. Stern, Center for Veterinary Health Sciences, Oklahoma State University, Stillwater, OK; [*B*] *Courtesy* Dr S.D. Cramer, Center for Veterinary Health Sciences, Oklahoma State University, Stillwater, OK.)

Intestines

In health, intestines vary from pale pink to purple when viewed from the serosal surface and pink-purple to red when the mucosal surface is examined. The mucosal surface has a moist to very wet, velvety, glistening sheen, analogous to a glossy paint finish. Throughout its length, there are mucosal folds designed to increase surface area. Moving aborally, villi tend to decrease in length with no villi present in the large intestine, whereas goblet cell numbers increase such that they are maximal in the distal large intestine.

In general, enteritis is a relatively pedestrian diagnosis histologically but can be very confusing grossly. Redness is only one feature to consider when determining if an animal has enteritis, given that in many cases mucosal redness is a variation of normal. Gross evidence of enteritis is reliably identifiable when there is adherent ingesta mixed with fibrin, erosions, ulcers, and mural necrosis (**Fig. 42**). Other features include luminal casts of necrotic material and mucosal thickening without loss of the mucosal sheen. Serosal changes to look for include mural edema, serosal congestion or multifocal hemorrhage (**Fig. 43**), loss of the normal serosal glistening surface, and adherent

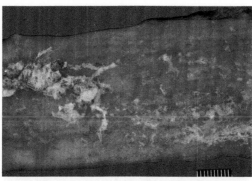

Fig. 42. Enteritis. The mucosal surface of this small intestinal section lacks the normal velvety, glistening sheen and instead is dull, partially covered by fibrin mixed with feed material, and has multifocal areas of mucosal hemorrhage. (*Courtesy* Dr R.J. Panciera, Center for Veterinary Health Sciences, Oklahoma State University, Stillwater, OK.)

fibrin. If serosal fibrin is mixed with feed material a perforation must be suspected. Finally, enteritis typically results in abnormal fluid contents downstream in the large intestine.

Bright red intestinal mucosa caused by hemorrhage with luminal necrotic debris or clotted blood is in indication of enteritis (**Fig. 44**). In general, causes to consider include *Eimeria* spp; coronavirus (winter dysentery); BVDV; MCF; *Clostridium* spp; heavy metal intoxication; *Salmonella* spp; bowel strangulations; and *Trichuris* spp (whipworms).[3,11] When large amounts of fibrin are present overlying the mucosal surface, causes to consider include *Salmonella* spp or *Clostridium* spp (**Fig. 45**). If there is hemorrhage and necrosis of the Peyer's patches or regional lymphoid tissue, BVD, *Salmonella* spp, or both should be strongly considered as possible causes for this lesion (**Fig. 46**).[11] Chronically, salmonellosis can manifest as focal areas of necrosis rimmed by fibrosis, commonly referred to a "button ulcers"

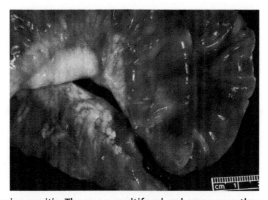

Fig. 43. Hemorrhagic serositis. There are multifocal red areas over the serosa representing areas of mural hemorrhage and necrosis. This same injury could be observed from the mucosal surface indicating evidence for enteritis. (*Courtesy* Indiana Animal Disease Diagnostic Laboratory, Purdue University, West Lafayette, IN.)

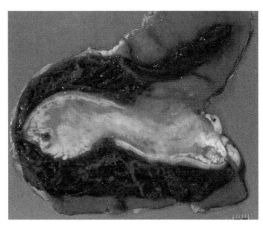

Fig. 44. Hemorrhagic enteritis. The intestinal mucosa is red and congested with large mats of blood clots mixed with fibrin strands and feed material. This lesion has several potential causes but in this case is an example of coccidiosis. (*Courtesy* Dr R.J. Panciera, Center for Veterinary Health Sciences, Oklahoma State University, Stillwater, OK.)

(**Fig. 47**).[11] Intestinal contents tend to have a more putrid, pungent odor caused by the amount of miasma present in cases of some bacterial enteritis, such as salmonellosis.

Mycobacterium avium subspecies *paratuberculosis*, the causative organism for Johne's disease, is a resilient intracellular organism that induces a prominent granulomatous reaction. Large numbers of macrophages are attracted to the lamina propria and submucosa of the affected intestine resulting in distinctive corrugation of the mucosa (**Fig. 48**) with a subsequent reduction in luminal diameter and functional absorptive surface area. In addition, a distinctive serosal and mesenteric response to this organism is granulomatous lymphangitis (see **Fig. 48**B).

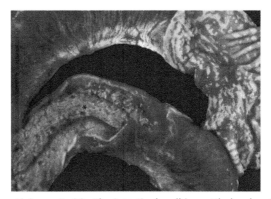

Fig. 45. Fibrinonecrotizing enteritis. The intestinal wall is mottled red and tan. The mucosa has lost is typical velvety sheen and is overlayed by a mat of fibrin. There is a large luminal clot of fibrin (*asterisk*). This lesion was caused by *Clostridium perfringens*. (*Courtesy* Indiana Animal Disease Diagnostic Laboratory, Purdue University, West Lafayette, IN.)

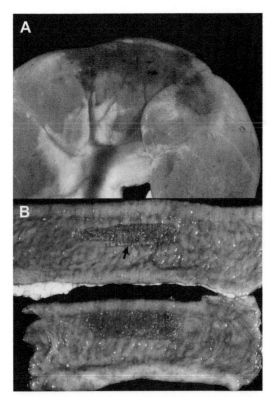

Fig. 46. Peyer's patch necrosis caused by BVD. (*A*) Along the antimesenteric edge of this section of small intestine is an area of necrosis and hemorrhage that corresponds to Peyer's patches. (*B*) Mucosal surface of small intestine depicting necrosis of Peyer's patches (*arrow*) with adherent fibrin and necrotic debris. This lesion is typical for BVDV infections. ([*A*] *Courtesy* Indiana Animal Disease Diagnostic Laboratory, Purdue University, West Lafayette, IN; [*B*] *Courtesy* Dr R.J. Panciera, Center for Veterinary Health Sciences, Oklahoma State University, Stillwater, OK.)

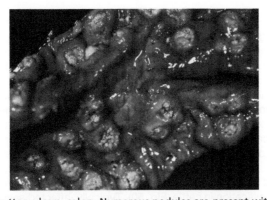

Fig. 47. Chronic button ulcers, colon. Numerous nodules are present with raised, rounded edges and central regions of necrosis. These lesions are a mucosal response to chronic *Salmonella* spp infection, which was confirmed in this case. (*Courtesy* Dr B.L. Njaa, Center for Veterinary Health Sciences, Oklahoma State University, Stillwater, OK.)

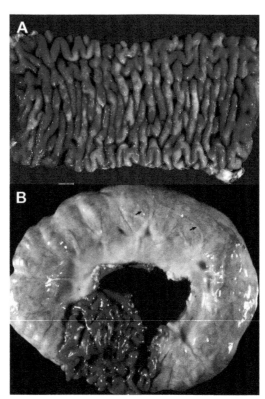

Fig. 48. Granulomatous ileitis. (*A*) An opened section of small intestine with a proliferative, corrugated appearance. This lesions is virtually pathognomonic for Johne's disease in cattle. (*B*) Partially opened section of small intestine with a similarly proliferative mucosa. Additionally, there are serosal lymphatics that are prominent because of a granulomatous lymphangitis (*arrows*), a more subtle lesion also typical for Johne's disease. ([*A*] *Courtesy* Dr R.J. Panciera, Center for Veterinary Health Sciences, Oklahoma State University, Stillwater, OK; [*B*] *Courtesy* Dr C.G. Lamm, College of Veterinary Medicine, Cornell University, Ithaca, NY.)

Jejunal hemorrhagic syndrome (or hemorrhagic bowel syndrome) is a relatively poorly understood entity of cattle resulting from chronic and ongoing intraluminal small intestinal hemorrhage without any evidence of concurrent enteritis (**Fig. 49**). Typically, affected animals present with signs of obstruction or possibly sudden death. The lesion can be segmental with variably sized collections of clotted blood that tend to minimally distend affected loops and yet have an underlying mucosa that is typically grossly normal. Isolation of *Clostridium perfringens* type A from cattle with this condition has been reported but likely does not represent a definitive cause.[17] Others have reported in dairy cattle that intensive management procedures and minimal exposure to pasture in high producing herds are predisposing factors to the development of this syndrome.[18]

Mesenteric and omental fat and other fat stores can become massively necrotic with areas of saponification in cattle (**Fig. 50**). Typically, affected animals are overconditioned, 2 years of age or older, and frequently of Channel Island lineage. The areas of necrosis and saponification are palpably hard and potentially obstructive. These lesions can vary from incidental findings to a cause of intestinal obstruction.[11]

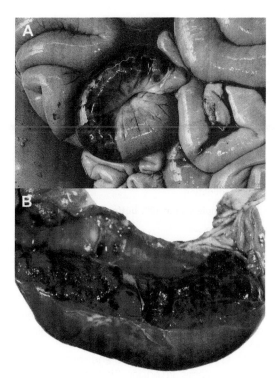

Fig. 49. Jejunal hemorrhagic syndrome. (*A*) Unopened loops of small intestine, focally hemorrhagic and mildly dilated because of a luminal blood clot. These luminal blood clots tend to lodge and obstruct. (*B*) Opened segment of small intestine with luminal clots of blood but a mucosal surface that appears grossly normal. ([*A*] *Courtesy* Dr F. Uzal, California Animal Health and Food Safety Laboratory, University of California, Davis, CA; [*B*] *Courtesy* College of Veterinary Medicine, Cornell University, Ithaca, NY.)

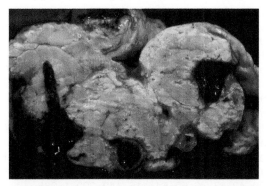

Fig. 50. Massive omental fat necrosis. This is a lesion that occurs most commonly in Channel Island cattle. Lesions vary from clinically incidental to obstructive. The necrotic fat is typically saponified and palpably hard. (*Courtesy* College of Veterinary Medicine, Cornell University, Ithaca, NY.)

Sample collection for gastrointestinal disease

- Gastrointestinal tissues autolyze rapidly after death. Therefore, a short postmortem interval is paramount and samples should be collected early in the necropsy procedure
- For remote necropsies, a few clear digital images of the gross lesions is very helpful when interpreting the case
- Collect samples for microbiologic testing first
  - Isolate the bowel segments for submission and tie off with string to keep contents intraluminal
  - Keep gastrointestinal samples separate from other tissue samples when submitting or shipping samples to a diagnostic laboratory
- Samples for histologic examination
  - Multiple tissues from multiple sites in 10% buffered formalin
  - Lesional and nonlesional tissues
  - Ensure that luminal and serosal surfaces are adequately bathed with formalin

---

REFERENCES

1. Schummer A, Nickel R, Sack WO. The alimentary canal of the ruminants. In: The viscera of the domestic mammals. 2nd revised edition. New York: Springer-Verlag; 1979. p. 148, 168.
2. Dyce KM, Sack WO, Wensing CJ. The head and ventral neck of the ruminants. In: Textbook of veterinary anatomy. 3rd edition. Philadelphia: Saunders; 2002. p. 636–7.
3. Helman RG. Interpretation of basic gross pathologic changes of the digestive tract. Vet Clin North Am Food Anim Pract 2000;16:1–22.
4. Thompson K. Bones and joints. In: Maxie MG, editor. Jubb, Kennedy, and Palmer's Pathology of domestic animals, vol. 1, 5th edition. Elsevier; 2007. p. 98–9.
5. Brown CC, Baker DC, Barker IK. Alimentary System. In: Maxie MG, editor. Jubb, Kennedy, and Palmer's Pathology of domestic animals, vol. 2, 5th edition. Elsevier; 2007. p. 20–1.
6. Masuda EK, Kommers GD, Martins TB, et al. Morphologic factors as indicators of malignancy of squamous cell carcinomas in cattle exposed naturally to bracken fern (Pteridium aquilium). J Comp Pathol 2011;144:48–54.
7. Radostits OM, Gay CC, Hinchcliff KW, et al. Diseases of the alimentary tract - II. In: Veterinary medicine: a textbook of the diseases of cattle, horses, sheep, pigs, and goats. Saunders Elsevier; 2007. p. 325–36.
8. Soulsby EJ. Nematodes. In: Helminths, arthropods, protozoa of domesticated animals. 6th edition. Baltimore (MD): Williams and Wilkins; 1974. p. 281–3.
9. Bowman DD. Helminths. In: Georgis' parasitology for veterinarnians. 9th edition. St Louis (MO): Saunders Elsevier; 2009. p. 124, 211.
10. Munz E, Dumbell K. Bovine papular stomatitis. In: Coetzer JAW, Tustin RC, editors. Infections diseases of livestock, vol. 2, 2nd edition. South Africa: Oxford University Press; 2004. p. 1289–90.
11. Brown CC, Baker DC, Barker IK. Alimentary system. In: Maxie MG, editor. Jubb, Kennedy, and Palmer's pathology of domestic animals, vol. 2, 5th edition. Elsevier; 2007. p. 39, 42–43, 46–50, 54, 116, 142, 200–1, 285.
12. Konig HE, Liebich HG. Digestive system. In: Konig HE, Leibich H-G, editors. Veterinary anatomy of domestic mammals: textbook and colour atlas. 3rd edition. Stuttgart (Germany): Schattauer; 2007. p. 338–9.

13. Campbell JR. Effect of bovine viral diarrhea virus in the feedlot. Vet Clin North Am Food Anim Pract 2004;20:39–50.
14. Teixeira AF, Kuhnel W, Vives P, et al. Functional morphology of unguiculiform papillae of the reticular groove of the ruminant stomach. Ann Anat 2009;191: 469–76.
15. Trent AM. Surgery of the abomasum. In: Fubini SL, Ducharme NG, editors. Farm animal surgery. St Louis (MO): Elsevier; 2004. p. 196–240.
16. Valli VE. Hematopoietic system. In: Maxie MG, editor. Jubb, Kennedy, and Palmer's pathology of domestic animals, vol. 3, 5th edition. Elsevier; 2007. p. 199–200.
17. Abutarbush SM, Radostits OM. Jejunal hemorrhage syndrome in diary and beef cattle: 11 cases (2001 to 2003). Can Vet J 2005;46:711–5.
18. Berghaus RD, McCluskey BJ, Callan RJ. Risk factors associated with hemorrhagic bowel syndrome in dairy cattle. J Am Vet Med Assoc 2005;226:1700–6.
19. Bielefeldt-Ohmann H. The pathologies of bovine viral diarrhea virus infection: a window on the pathogenesis. Vet Clin North Am Food Anim Pract 1995;11: 447–76.
20. Saliki JT, Dubovi EJ. Laboratory diagnosis of bovine viral diarrhea virus infections. Vet Clin North Am Food Anim Pract 2004;20:69–84.

Neuropathology and Diagnostics in Food Animals

Jerome C. Nietfeld, DVM, PhD

KEYWORDS

- Neuropathology • Diagnostics • Cattle • Sheep • Pigs • Food animals

KEY POINTS

- Diseases of the central nervous system (CNS) are relatively common in food animals; potential causes include infectious agents, nutritional deficiencies, metabolic disorders, genetic defects, toxins, and idiopathic causes.
- Knowing the age, sex, breed, intended use, and management of animals provides much valuable information because the differentials for neurologic diseases for neonates, juveniles, and adults are usually different.
- An antemortem diagnosis is preferable to a postmortem one because it allows for possible treatment of affected individuals, but that is often not possible.
- Determining the correct etiologic diagnosis often depends on a thorough postmortem examination, collection of samples and accurate interpretation of postmortem findings and laboratory tests.

Diseases of the central nervous system (CNS) are relatively common in food animals. Potential causes include infectious agents, nutritional deficiencies, metabolic disorders, genetic defects, toxins, and idiopathic causes. Food animals are frequently raised in large groups, there is often human and animal traffic between groups, and large numbers of animals are often fed the same ration. This situation makes an accurate and timely etiologic diagnosis important so that treatment can be initiated and the spread of infectious agents and toxins limited.

An antemortem diagnosis is preferable to a postmortem one because it allows for possible treatment of affected individuals, but this is not always possible. Determining the correct etiologic diagnosis often depends on a thorough postmortem examination and collection of samples. Critical components for making an accurate diagnosis are the gathering of as much information as possible, a thorough examination of affected and unaffected animals and their surroundings, performance of a thorough necropsy

The author has nothing to disclose.
Department of Diagnostic Medicine/Pathobiology, College of Veterinary Medicine, Kansas State University, Mosier Hall, 1800 Denison Avenue, Manhattan, KS 66506, USA
E-mail address: nietfeld@vet.k-state.edu

Vet Clin Food Anim 28 (2012) 515–534
http://dx.doi.org/10.1016/j.cvfa.2012.07.008
vetfood.theclinics.com

and collection of the appropriate diagnostic samples, and accurate interpretation of the diagnostic findings. The goals of this article are:

- To review some of the steps and procedures necessary to collect the necessary information
- To briefly describe a few techniques for examination of the CNS
- To review some of the gross pathology likely to be encountered in a food animal practice

SIGNALMENT AND HISTORY

Knowing the age, sex, breed, intended use, and management of animals provides much valuable information because the differentials for neurologic diseases for neonates, juveniles, and adults are usually different. Similarly, the differentials for cows at pasture are often different than those for dairy cattle. A 3-day-old calf is much more likely to have *Escherichia coli* meningitis than an adult dairy cow, whereas a dairy cow being fed corn silage is more likely to have listeriosis. Although calves in a feedlot and at pasture can develop polioencephalomalacia, the condition is more prevalent in feedlot calves.

As complete a history as possible and a thorough description of the problem as seen by the animals' caretaker are important. How long has the problem been going on? What are the major clinical signs? Are the clinical signs mild, severe, or intermediate when first noticed? Are animals found unexpectedly dead? Have any been treated? Do they improve with time or treatment? How large is the group? What is the morbidity and mortality? Is the situation improving, static, or worsening? Do affected animals continue to eat and drink? These and other questions will often provide valuable clues as to whether the problem is neurologic or referable to another system, and give insight into potential causes. For instance, knowing that a young goat with severe paresis or paralysis of the rear legs (**Fig. 1**) has been steadily becoming more ataxic and weaker for several weeks leads one to suspect caprine arthritis-encephalomyelitis, whereas spinal trauma is more likely if the goat was normal yesterday. Knowing that calves with acute neurologic symptoms that include blindness and are suspected of having

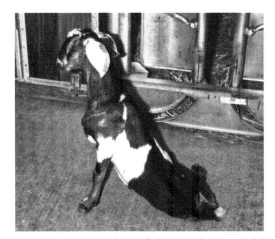

Fig. 1. A young goat with paresis/paralysis of the rear legs caused by caprine arthritis-encephalomyelitis (CAE) virus. Clinically, trauma to the vertebral column and spinal cord could cause the same symptoms.

polioencephalomalacia have not responded to thiamine treatment should make one suspect lead poisoning.

EXAMINATION OF LIVING ANIMALS

A neurologic examination combined with a thorough history will usually allow the clinician to determine whether a problem is due to disease of the CNS or another organ system, and will help localize the problem. Although many procedures used to examine small animals and horses are often not possible with food animals, protocols for safe examination of food animals have been described.[1,2] In some cases the diagnosis will be made on the basis of the clinical examination and history. Tetanus is a good example. Diagnostic tests to identify tetanus toxin are rarely available, isolation is usually not attempted or is negative, and there are no pathologic lesions. Diagnosis is almost always based on clinical signs that include stiffness, tonic spasms, and hyperesthesia, which progress to lateral recumbency and generalized tetanic spasms with the head thrown back and the limbs rigid. This holds particularly true if the animal has a history of surgery, wounds, or giving birth in the past few weeks (**Fig. 2**A). It is important to rule out other possible diseases such as bacterial meningitis, which can clinically resemble tetanus and follows surgical procedures and wounds (see **Fig. 2**B).

Serum and whole blood should be collected and saved; they may not be needed, but often blood and/or serum will be useful or necessary for making a diagnosis. For instance, cerebral hypoxia caused by anaplasmosis (or other causes of severe acute anemia) and hypocalcemia can cause aggression in cattle, and the diagnosis of both is difficult without serum or blood. Hepatic encephalopathy, hypomagnesemic tetany in ruminants, and hypoglycemia in neonatal pigs are additional examples of diseases with neurologic signs whereby serum is helpful or necessary for an accurate diagnosis. Whole blood as well as hair and skin are often used to identify heterozygous and homozygous carriers of many inherited diseases, such as α- and β-mannosidosis in various breeds of cattle and Nubian goats, and arthrogryposis multiplex in Angus calves.

Cerebrospinal fluid (CSF) can provide useful information, and techniques for safe collection from the lumbosacral space, processing, examination, and interpretation of results have been described.[3] CSF analysis is most useful for diagnosis of infectious diseases as opposed to noninfectious toxic, metabolic, and degenerative diseases in which the CSF characteristics are often normal.[3,4] Acute bacterial infections, such as neonatal meningitis and thrombotic meningoencephalitis (TME) caused by *Histophilus somni* (*Haemophilus somnus*), are typically accompanied by a neutrophilic pleocytosis,[3,4] and often an etiologic diagnosis can be made by bacterial culture. Chronic bacterial diseases, such as listeriosis, abscesses, and viral diseases tend to be

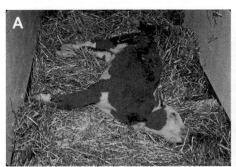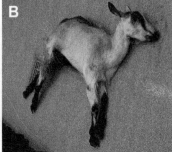

Fig. 2. (*A*) Calf with tetanus. (*B*) Kid with bacterial meningitis.

accompanied by mononuclear pleocytosis.[4] The usual recommendation is that cytologic examination of CSF samples should be done within 2 hours of collection.[3] A recent study found no significant differences between total and differential cell counts in CSF samples from calves using split samples examined within 1 hour and 24 hours after collection when the 24-hour samples were stored at 4°C after adding 11% autologous serum.[5]

POSTMORTEM EXAMINATION
Examine and Collect Samples from Entire Animal

In many cases animals are found dead, they die despite treatment, they are euthanized for humane reasons, or it is more economical to euthanize them. It is then necessary to perform a necropsy and collect samples to support or make a diagnosis. Multiple procedures for performing food animal necropsies have been published and are not reviewed here.[6-11] Even in cases where clinical signs point to neurologic disease, it is important to thoroughly examine and sample the entire animal because some neurologic diseases cannot be diagnosed by examination of the CNS. Sample collection should be done with the idea that it is better to save a sample and not need it than to later wish it had been saved. **Table 1** lists some diagnostic characteristics of infectious diseases that are not primary CNS infections, metabolic and toxic diseases in which there are neurologic symptoms, but for which examination of nonneural samples is necessary or helpful in making the correct diagnosis. **Table 2** lists primary infectious diseases of the CNS and samples required for diagnosis.

CSF can often be collected while disarticulating the head at the atlanto-occipital joint.[10] Incise the tissues covering the ventral surface of the joint, including the atlanto-occipital membrane, and insert a needle attached to a syringe through the dura mater until hitting bone. Withdraw the needle slightly and aspirate (**Fig. 3**). If the needle is inserted off midline, the likelihood of aspirating blood is decreased. The CSF should be clear, and cloudiness suggests bacterial infection. Blood could be from antemortem hemorrhage, but is more likely from puncturing a vein during collection. In suspected cases of bacterial meningitis, CSF is an excellent sample for bacterial culture.

Always remove and save unfixed and fixed tonsils of pigs because they are a preferred sample for many diseases, such as pseudorabies, *Teschovirus* (*Enterovirus*), classic swine fever, African swine fever, porcine reproductive and respiratory syndrome virus, and porcine circovirus type 2. Similarly, remove and save the retropharyngeal lymph nodes of sheep, goats, and cervids, because they and the obex are used for diagnosis of scrapie in sheep and goats and chronic wasting disease in cervids (**Fig. 4**).

If hypomagnesemic tetany is possible, remove the eyes and either collect the vitreous humor or save the entire eye for magnesium analysis. Concentrations of Mg in serum, CSF, aqueous humor, and vitreous humor are related in living cattle, but after death the concentration is not stable in serum, CSF, or aqueous humor, but is stable in the vitreous humor.[12,13] Magnesium concentrations of 0.55 mmol/L (1.3 mg/dL) or less in the vitreous humor of adult cattle are diagnostic of hypomagnesemia for up to 48 hours after death.[12,13] Similarly, Mg concentrations of 0.65 mmol/L (1.6 mg/dL) or less in the vitreous humor of adult sheep are diagnostic for up to 24 hours after death.[13] Ocular fluid is also often used to diagnose nitrate toxicity.

Removal of the Brain and Collection of Samples for Rabies and Transmissible Spongiform Encephalopathies

With only a little practice, brains can be removed quickly and safely. Probably the simplest method is to cut the skull lengthwise on the midline with a saw and remove the brain from the respective halves (**Fig. 5**). The brain can also be removed intact with a hatchet, axe, cleaver, chisel and mallet, or hand saw.[6–11] It is important to closely examine the brain, the bones of the calvaria, and the meninges for fractures, hemorrhages, tumors and other space-occupying lesions, purulent exudate, and other abnormalities.

If rabies is a possibility, it is critical that the correct samples be collected and properly submitted to the laboratory. In the past, a common recommendation was to split the brain lengthwise and submit half fresh and half in 10% buffered formalin.[14] This guideline is no longer acceptable, because the Centers for Disease Control and Prevention require that a complete cross section of brainstem and either the cerebellum or the hippocampuses, with the cerebellum preferred, be tested for a brain to be reported as negative.[15] The preferred sample is a transverse section through the cerebellum and the underlying brainstem submitted unfixed, either frozen or unfrozen (**Fig. 6**). If the brain is split lengthwise, submit sections from both halves of the brainstem and cerebellum. In ruminants, remove the brainstem section for rabies anterior to the obex and save the obex to be tested for transmissible spongiform encephalopathies (TSE): scrapie, chronic wasting disease, or bovine spongiform encephalopathy (see **Fig. 6**). After saving samples for rabies and TSE tests, one can save the remainder of the brain as wished.

Removal and Examination of the Spinal Cord

The spinal cord is more difficult and time consuming to examine and remove. Consequently, it is not examined in some cases where it would be helpful or necessary to make a definitive diagnosis. Realistically it is not necessary to remove the spinal cord in all cases where there is evidence of spinal cord involvement. If one finds evidence of lymphoma in lymph nodes and organs of a down, alert cow and concludes that lymphoma involving the spinal canal is the cause of recumbency without opening the canal, one will rarely be wrong. Careful examination of the outer surfaces of vertebral bodies will often reveal fractures or abscesses that are the cause of paresis and paralysis, making cord removal unnecessary (**Fig. 7**).

In cases of diffuse CNS involvement, such as viral or bacterial infections, the diagnosis can usually be made by examination of only brain or brain plus sections of the spinal cord. However, there are infectious diseases for which examination of the spinal cord is important. For example, in species other than pigs, such as cattle, pseudorabies virus infection is often by the oral route and the virus follows autonomic nerves from the intestines to the spinal cord to the brain. Sometimes animals die before detectable virus reaches the brain, and the spinal cord must be tested to identify pseudorabies virus. However, a few small pieces of spinal cord are as good as the entire cord. Make transverse cuts through the vertebral column and remove sections about 2 vertebrae in length (**Fig. 8A**). Swab the subdural space and save for bacterial culture. Using a pair of thin scissors and small tweezers, cut the nerve rootlets and remove the pieces of cord (see **Fig. 8B**).

Sometimes the entire cord or large portions of the cord need to be examined, usually to find localized lesions such as fractures or abscesses. Another example is selenium toxicity in pigs whereby the lesions are usually restricted to the gray matter of the cervicothoracic and lumbar enlargements. Removing the entire cord is more work than removing a few pieces, but it can be done in the field. In neonatal animals, such as pigs, sheep, and goats, the cord can be exposed by removing the dorsal arches with diagonal pliers purchased at a hardware store (**Fig. 9**). The cord of calves up to 150 to 200 kg, juvenile goats and sheep, and nursery/finishing pigs can be exposed in only a few minutes with a hand saw by laying the animal on its side,

Table 1
Diagnosis of secondary, metabolic, and toxic neurologic diseases

Disease/Condition	Primary Lesions	Lesions in CNS	Diagnosis
Nervous coccidiosis in calves	Spiral colon	None	1. Clinical signs 2. Identify coccidial infection 3. Rule out primary CNS disease
Edema disease in pigs	Edema of brain, Stomach, mesocolon, eyelids	Microscopic: vascular necrosis, edema, focal malacia	1. Isolation of Shiga toxin producing *Escherichia coli* from small intestine 2. Acute CNS signs and typical lesions
Enterotoxemia–*Clostridium perfringens* type D	Pericardial effusion, visceral hemorrhages, glucosuria	Focal symmetric hemorrhage and malacia	1. Identify toxin in intestinal contents 2. Isolate *C perfringens* type D from intestines 3. Microscopic lesions in brain
Tetanus–*Clostridium tetani*	Infected wound; often no lesion	None	1. Clinical signs—most common 2. Isolation of *C tetani* from wound
Botulism—*Clostridium botulinum*	Ingestion of *C botulinum* toxin	None	1. Clinical signs 2. Identify toxin in serum
Lead toxicity–ruminants	Cerebrum	Usually no lesions Laminar necrosis possible	Determination of lead levels in: 1. Whole blood 2. Kidney 3. Liver (kidney is preferred)
Sodium toxicity due to water deprivation—pigs	Cerebrum	Laminar necrosis, eosinophilic inflammation	1. Brain Na levels 2. Histologic lesions in brain 3. Serum and CSF Na
Sodium toxicity due to excess Na intake	Uncertain	None (sometimes laminar necrosis)	1. Brain Na levels 2. Serum or CSF Na levels

Hypomagnesemic tetany—ruminants	None	None	1. Serum or plasma Mg levels—antemortem 2. Vitreous humor Mg levels—postmortem
Hypocalcemia	None	None	1. Serum Ca—antemortem only
Hypoglycemia—neonatal pigs, ketosis, pregnancy toxemia	None	None	1. History 2. Hypoglycemia 3. Ketones in urine
Vitamin A deficiency	Membranous bones	Dorsoventral compression of brain, coning and herniation of cerebellum	1. Clinical signs—blindness, convulsions 2. Gross lesions 3. Vitamin A measurement—definitive
Anaplasmosis	Anemia resulting in cerebral hypoxia	None	1. Verify anemia 2. Identify parasite in blood smear 3. Serum ELISA or PCR of whole blood
Organophosphate and carbamate toxicity	None	None	1. Whole blood cholinesterase level 2. Brain cholinesterase level 3. Identification of agent in stomach/rumen contents, tissues, and/or source
Selenium toxicity in pigs	Separation at coronary band of hooves	Necrosis in ventral horns of spinal cord	Selenium levels in blood, serum, or tissues
Nonprotein nitrogen toxicity	Excessive ammonia released in gastrointestinal tract and hyperammonemia	Microscopic: spongy degeneration of white matter is possible	1. Rumen pH >7.5–8 at time of death 2. Measurement of ammonia levels in rumen contents, serum, blood—must be within 12 h of death or 2 h in hot weather

Abbreviations: ELISA, enzyme-linked immunosorbent assay; PCR, polymerase chain reaction.

Table 2
Diagnosis of infectious causes of neurologic disease

Disease/Condition	Primary Lesions	Lesions in CNS	Diagnosis
Bacterial meningitis/ encephalomyelitis	Meninges, brain, spinal cord	Suppurative meningitis	1. Bacterial culture of meninges, brain, CSF 2. Histologic examination of brain
Thrombotic encephalomyelitis	1. Brain 2. Joints 3. Heart	Hemorrhages, thrombosis, suppurative inflammation	1. Gross and histologic lesions 2. Isolation of *Histophilus somni*
Listeriosis	Brainstem	Microabscesses and perivascular lymphocytic cuffing	1. Histologic lesions 2. Immunohistochemical staining 3. Isolation of *Listeria* spp
Viral diseases, ie, rabies, West Nile virus, herpesviruses	Brain, spinal cord	Nonsuppurative encephalitis, encephalomyelitis (occasionally suppurative)	1. Identification of causative virus
Caprine arthritis-encephalomyelitis, ovine progressive pneumonia	Spinal cord, brain, synovial membranes, lungs, mammary glands	Nonsuppurative encephalomyelitis, patchy demyelination	1. Clinical signs coupled with microscopic changes in spinal cord and brain—cord lesions most characteristic 2. Presence of serum antibodies 3. Virus identification by PCR (least common method)
Congenital viral infections	Brain, spinal cord, other tissues	Hydranencephaly, cerebellar hypoplasia, microphthalmia, and so forth	1. Identification of causative virus 2. Presence of precolostral antibodies

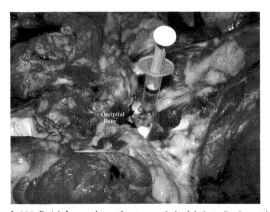

Fig. 3. Collection of CSF fluid from the atlanto-occipital joint. By inserting the needle off center, the likelihood of aspirating blood is decreased.

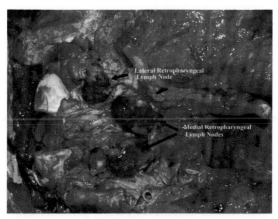

Fig. 4. Retropharyngeal lymph nodes are used to test for scrapie in sheep and goats, and for chronic wasting disease in cervids. Note that the left lateral retropharyngeal node has been removed.

removing the limbs and ribs from the up side, and cutting parallel to the dorsal processes just off midline, opening the spinal canal while taking care to not cut into the cord (**Fig. 10**). This technique is especially helpful in examining young animals for pathology such as vertebral fractures, abscesses, meningitis, and vertebral malformations. Opening the spinal canal of larger animals such as juvenile and adult cattle and adult swine can be accomplished with an axe by cutting away the lateral portions of the vertebrae (**Fig. 11**). It is messy and can be considerable work, but it takes little, if any, longer to expose the cord with an axe than with a band saw. Once the cord is exposed, examine the vertebrae and intervertebral disks and remove the cord by grasping the dura mater with a forceps and cutting the nerve rootlets. Open the dura with scissors, swab the subdural space, remove a few pieces of fresh cord for bacterial and viral testing, and fix the remainder in formalin.

GROSS PATHOLOGY OF THE BRAIN AND SPINAL CORD
Meningitis, Encephalitis, and Meningoencephalitis

Cloudiness and purulent exudates on the meningeal surfaces indicate bacterial meningitis, which is more likely in young animals than in adults (**Fig. 12**). Bacterial

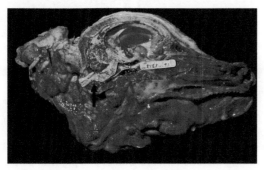

Fig. 5. Head from a calf with hydrocephalus that has been split lengthwise on the midline. Note the acute, upward deviation of the brainstem (*arrow*), which restricts flow of CSF, resulting in hydrocephalus.

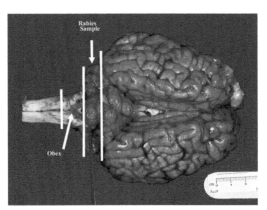

Fig. 6. Brain from a calf. Vertical lines indicates where to cut to obtain samples for rabies and transmissible spongiform encephalopathy (TSE) tests. A section through the cerebellum and underlying brainstem (*right arrow*) is the preferred sample for rabies, and the obex (*left arrow*) is necessary for TSE tests.

meningitis is a systemic disease, and finding fibrinopurulent arthritis and polyserositis in a young animal should alert one to the possibility of meningitis. Hemorrhages on the outer or cut surfaces of cattle brains, especially feedlot cattle, indicate thrombotic meningoencephalitis (thromboembolic meningoencephalitis or TEME) caused by *Histophilus somni* (**Fig. 13**). Cloudy joint fluid and CSF, and hemorrhages in the heart of feedlot cattle suggest that *H somni* infection of the brain is likely (**Fig. 14**). Swollen thin-walled lateral ventricles and swellings, and soft spots in other areas of the brain can represent an abscess, hemorrhage, hydrocephalus, or tumor (**Fig. 15**).

Listeriosis of ruminants affects the brainstem, but is usually not accompanied by macroscopic lesions. Bacterial isolation is often unsuccessful, and diagnosis is most commonly by identification of characteristic microabscesses in histologic sections of brainstem. In the author's experience, identification of *Listeria* spp by immunohistochemical staining of formalin-fixed brain is more often successful than is bacterial culture. The 2 most important differentials for listeriosis are otitis media/interna and a brainstem abscess, which can be eliminated at necropsy. Also, animals with otitis are typically alert and do not have nystagmus.[2,16]

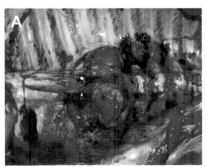
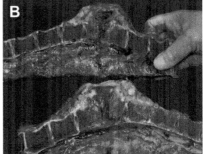

Fig. 7. Abscesses involving thoracic vertebral bodies of a pig with paralysis of the rear legs. In (*A*) the abscesses bulge into the thoracic cavity, alleviating the need to open the spinal canal to determine the cause of the paralysis. In (*B*) the vertebral bodies have been sectioned with a handsaw to demonstrate the extent of involvement.

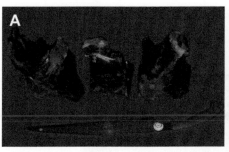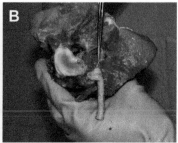

Fig. 8. (*A*) Sections of spinal column from a feeder calf removed with a handsaw. (*B*) The spinal cord is removed by cutting the nerve rootlets with a small scissors and retracting the cord with a forceps. Portions of each section of cord can be submitted fresh and formalin-fixed.

Enterotoxemia (overeating disease, pulpy kidney disease) caused by *Clostridium perfringens* type D in young lambs and calves is sometimes accompanied by neurologic signs that can include ataxia, head pressing, blindness, and convulsions. In subacute cases there often are bilaterally symmetric areas of hemorrhage and/or yellow discoloration in the midbrain and brainstem, which represent necrosis caused by toxin absorbed from the intestines.[17,18] In many cases, the necrosis is only visible microscopically, and it is only pathologic change that is considered diagnostic for enterotoxemia. Diagnosis can also be by identification of epsilon toxin in the intestinal contents or isolation of *C perfringens* type D from the intestines and glucosuria.

Viral infections typically cause nonsuppurative encephalitis or encephalomyelitis, but gross pathology is rare. Both formalin-fixed and unfixed brain, spinal cord, and other tissues are important for diagnosis. Even in cases where the virus is identified in neurologic tissues, it is helpful to examine the CNS for inflammation.

Hydrocephalus and Hydranencephaly

Hydrocephalus and hydranencephaly are relatively common, especially in neonatal food animals. Hydrocephalus is an increased volume of CSF in the cranial cavity

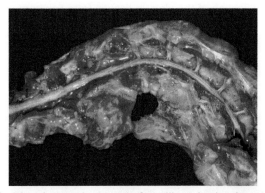

Fig. 9. Spinal cord within the vertebral canal of a stillborn lamb infected in utero by Cache Valley virus. The cord was exposed by removing the dorsal arches with diagonal pliers. Note the small size of the spinal cord in comparison with the spinal canal; normally, the spinal cord fills the spinal canal. This lamb was also affected by severe hydranencephaly, and its brain is shown in **Fig. 17**A.

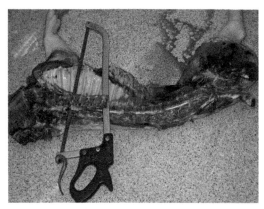

Fig. 10. Removing the spinal cord from a pig with a hand saw. The technique also works well for examination and removal of the spinal cord of young calves.

caused by restriction of circulation of the CSF or CSF filling spaces normally occupied by tissue that failed to develop. In food animals, only internal hydrocephalus with accumulation of CSF in the ventricles is common, and it is usually secondary to defects that restrict normal flow of CSF (see **Fig. 5**; **Fig. 16**).[17] Hydranencephaly is due to necrosis of developing cerebral tissue with accumulation of CSF in the resulting cavities (**Fig. 17**). It can vary from almost complete destruction of the cerebrum leaving only a CSF-filled sac (see **Fig. 17**A) to small fluid-filled holes in the cerebrum, referred to as porencephaly (see **Fig. 17**B).

Hydranencephaly is most commonly the result of in utero viral infection. In North America, viral causes include Cache Valley and Border disease (BD) viruses in sheep, bluetongue virus in sheep and cattle, and bovine viral diarrhea (BVD) virus in calves.[14,17,18] Worldwide, other viral causes of hydranencephaly include Akabane, Rift Valley fever, and Wesselsbron viruses in calves and sheep, and Chuzan virus in calves.[14,17,18] Since November 2011, a virus provisionally named Schmallenberg virus in the genus *Orthobunyavirus*, which includes Cache Valley and Akabane viruses, has been associated with outbreaks of hydranencephaly and scoliosis in sheep, goats, and cattle in Germany, Belgium, and the Netherlands.[19] Diagnosis of in utero viral infection is by identification of the virus in tissues from newborn or aborted animals

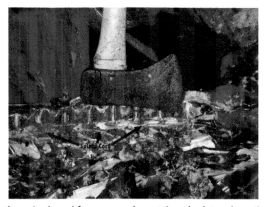

Fig. 11. Removing the spinal cord from a cow by cutting the lateral portions of the vertebral bodies with an axe.

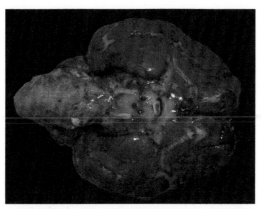

Fig. 12. Cloudy, greenish exudates on the ventral surface of a calf brain with bacterial meningitis.

or by detection of virus-specific antibody in serum obtained before ingestion of colostrum. In utero copper deficiency (congenital swayback) is a noninfectious cause of hydranencephaly in lambs and kids.[17,18,20]

Congenital hydrocephalus occurs in all food animal species and can be inherited as an autosomal recessive trait in multiple breeds of calves and, possibly, pigs.[17,18,20] Other causes of congenital hydrocephalus include the viral causes of hydranencephaly, ingestion of *Veratrum californicum* by pregnant sheep and cattle, and vitamin A deficiency in cattle because of defective absorption of CSF by the arachnoid.[17,18,20,21] Postnatal hydrocephalus can result from vitamin A deficiency in cattle and CNS inflammation in all species.[17] Vitamin A deficiency in fetal and growing animals, especially calves and piglets, also impairs growth of membranous bones that can result in compression of the brain and optic nerves leading to stillbirths, blindness, ataxia, and seizures.[21,22] At necropsy the optic canal is narrowed and there is compression of the brain with the cerebrum flattened and the cerebellum compressed, and sometimes herniated, into the foramen magnum (**Fig. 18**).

CEREBELLAR PATHOLOGY

Cerebellar hypoplasia is the failure of the cerebellum to develop fully (**Fig. 19**). The clinical signs are evident at birth, and it is a relatively common congenital anomaly that

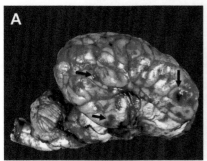
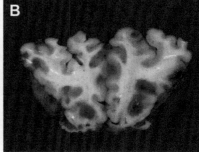

Fig. 13. Multiple hemorrhages on the outer surface (*A; arrows*) and cut surface (*B*) of a feedlot calf with thrombotic meningoencephalitis caused by *Histophilus somni*. (*Courtesy of* Drs Gordon Andrews and Giselle Cino Ozuna.)

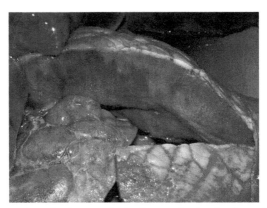

Fig. 14. Acute hemorrhage in the ventricular free wall of a feedlot calf with thrombotic meningoencephalitis caused by systemic *H somni* infection. This lesion is frequently seen in calves with CNS involvement.

occurs in all animal species. The condition can be inherited in Hereford, Shorthorn, Ayrshire, and Angus calves, and occurs in piglets whose dams were treated during pregnancy with the organophosphate insecticide trichlorofon.[17,18,23] Possibly the most common cause is viral infection at a stage of gestation when the cerebellum is growing rapidly. The most important causes are BVD virus in calves, BD virus in lambs, and classic swine fever virus in piglets.[17,18,20] Hypomyelination of the CNS frequently accompanies cerebellar hypoplasia caused by both in utero viral infection and exposure of pregnant sows to trichlorofon, and is manifest as muscular tremors referred to as congenital tremors or myoclonia congenital.[17,18,23] Congenital tremors in pigs can also be caused by pseudorabies virus and can be inherited in a few breeds.

Cerebellar abiotrophy is the premature degeneration of the cerebellum, which causes clinical signs of cerebellar disease in animals that were normal at birth. The cerebellum is of normal size or slightly smaller than normal, and diagnosis is by microscopic demonstration of excessive degeneration and loss of Purkinje cells and other cells in the cerebellum. Although toxic causes, such as in utero exposure to locoweed and organophosphates, are sometimes suspected,[23] most cases are believed to be inherited.[17,23]

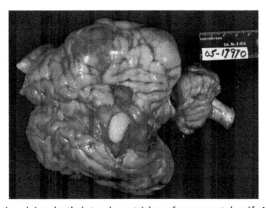

Fig. 15. Abscesses involving both lateral ventricles of a neonatal calf. Note the swellings involving the right cerebral cortex and the purulent exudates exuding from the incised left lateral ventricle.

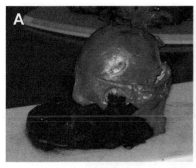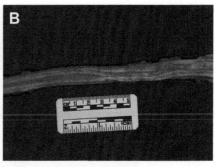

Fig. 16. Internal hydrocephalus in a calf resulting in doming of the cranium (A), which was caused by myelodysplasia with incomplete closure of the thoracolumbar spinal cord (B) and regional lack of the central canal.

Generalized cerebral swelling resulting from edema can cause rearward displacement and coning of the cerebellum owing to compression against the occipital bone (**Fig. 20**) and possibly herniation into the foramen magnum. Possible causes include bacterial encephalitis and/or meningitis, polioencephalomalacia, salt toxicity following water deprivation, and toxins such as lead and organomecuric compounds.[17] Arnold-Chiari malformation is an uncommon congenital anomaly that results in displacement of the posterior cerebellum through the foramen magnum into the first cervical vertebra, and is sometimes accompanied by spina bifida.[18]

LAMINAR CORTICAL NECROSIS OF THE CEREBRUM (POLIOENCEPHALOMALACIA)

Polioencephalomalacia of ruminants, sodium toxicity secondary to water deprivation in pigs, and lead poisoning in ruminants are characterized by similar clinical signs that include, but are not limited to, dullness, aimless wandering, head pressing, clonic convulsions, recumbency, and blindness. The lesions of polioencephalomalacia and water deprivation are cerebral edema and necrosis (malacia) of the outer lamina of gray matter of the cerebral cortex that sometimes can be seen as multifocal bands of yellow-brown discoloration.[17,18] Although the malacic areas are usually difficult to identify with certainty, when illuminated with a black light they glow and are easily

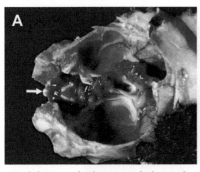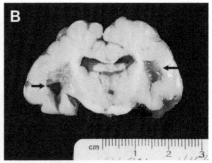

Fig. 17. (A) Severe hydranencephaly in a lamb infected in utero with Cache Valley virus. The cerebrum consisted of a thin, membranous sac filled with CSF, which ruptured when the skull was opened. The cerebellum is severely atrophied and the only relatively normal portion of the brain is the brainstem (*arrow*). (B) Porencephaly (*arrows*) in a lamb infected in utero with Cache Valley virus.

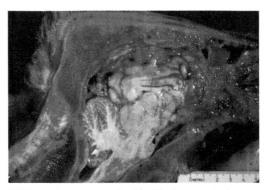

Fig. 18. Vitamin A deficiency in a neonatal calf with dorsoventral compression of the brain and rearward displacement of the cerebellum.

recognized (**Fig. 21**A, B). In pigs with water deprivation, laminar necrosis is typically accompanied by eosinophilic meningoencephalitis. Lead poisoning is sometimes listed as a cause of laminar necrosis, but the lesions are subtle and are usually not visible, even with a black light or microscopically. There is clinical evidence that sodium toxicity secondary to water deprivation can also cause laminar necrosis in ruminants, but this is proven only in pigs.[17] Sodium toxicity caused by ingestion of excess sodium can cause clinical signs of neurologic disease, but does not cause laminar necrosis, and the reason for the neurologic signs is unknown.[17]

SPINA BIFIDA, MYELODYSPLASIA, AND ARTHROGRYPOSIS

Myelodysplasia is abnormal development of the spinal cord and spina bifida is incomplete closure of the dorsal arches of one or more vertebrae, which usually affect the lumbosacral area (see **Fig. 16**B and **Fig. 22**A, C). The two conditions often occur together, but can occur independent of one another and are often accompanied by arthrogryposis (see **Fig. 22**B),[17] which can involve one or two limbs or be generalized. Arthrogryposis can result from lack of movement in utero, but denervation is more common and is often accompanied by hypoplasia of muscles.[17] The vertebral defect can be open so that the meninges are exposed (spina bifida cystica) (see **Fig. 22**A, C) or covered by skin so that the defect is not noticeable (spina bifida occulta). In cases of

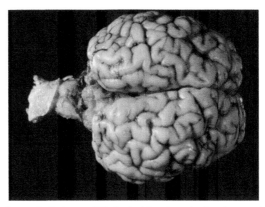

Fig. 19. Cerebellar hypoplasia in a calf infected in utero by bovine viral diarrhea virus.

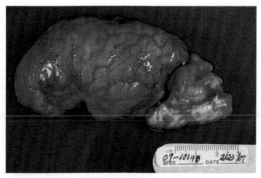

Fig. 20. Coning of the cerebellum of a calf brain caused by edema and rearward displacement against the occipital bone.

spina bifida occulta there usually is a small dimple at the location of the vertebral defect, and radiographs are the best method for diagnosis.

In North America, congenital arthrogryposis and muscular hypoplasia, often accompanied by hydranencephaly and spinal cord hypoplasia, occur in lambs infected in utero with Cache Valley virus (see **Figs. 9, 17; Fig. 23**). In other parts of the world, Akabane virus is an important cause of arthrogryposis and hydranencephaly in ruminants.[17] Bluetongue, BD, and BVD viruses are reported to cause arthrogryposis and hydranencephaly, but whereas brain malformations are relatively common, arthrogryposis is rare. Arthrogryposis can be inherited (eg, arthrogryposis multiplex of black Angus cattle), or be the result of ingestion of toxic plants by the mother during early gestation. Many cases are idiopathic.

OTHER CAUSES OF SPINAL CORD ABNORMALITY

The most common causes of abnormality of the spinal cord are vertebral fractures, abscesses, infections, and lymphoma in cattle. Bacterial and viral meningitis/myelitis are often not grossly visible, and diagnosis depends on histologic examination and identification of the causative agent. Occasionally areas of hemorrhage and yellowish

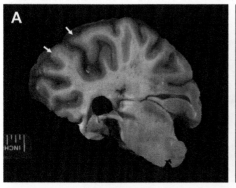
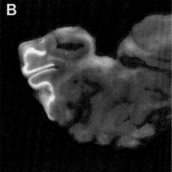

Fig. 21. Cross sections of cerebrum from calves with polioencephalomalacia. (*A*) The areas of yellow-brown necrosis involving the outer gray lamina of the cortex (*arrows*) can be difficult to identify with certainty. (*B*) Illumination with a black light makes the areas of laminar necrosis typical of polioencephalomalacia easily visible.

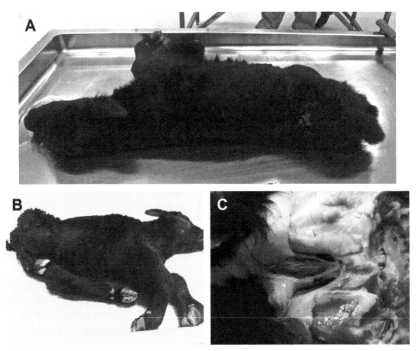

Fig. 22. Congenital spina bifida and arthrogryposis in a crossbred calf. (*A*) An open defect in the skin is present on the dorsal midline at the lumbosacral region. (*B*) Arthrogryposis affecting all 4 limbs. (*C*) The meningeal sac that protruded slightly through the skin and the vertebral defect has been incised to expose the spinal cord.

discoloration are visible in spinal cords from young goats with caprine arthritis-encephalomyelitis. Fractures can be diagnosed at necropsy or radiographically. Although other types of neoplasia can occur, lymphoma of the spinal canal of cattle is the only type that is important. Lymphoma can closely resemble fat, but fat floats in formalin and lymphoma does not. Ankylosing spondylosis is relatively common in older bulls and can result in acute paralysis. *Parelaphostrongylus tenuis* is a nematode that normally resides in the subarachnoid space of white-tailed deer. Occasionally the larvae migrate into the spinal cord of domestic ruminants, with South American

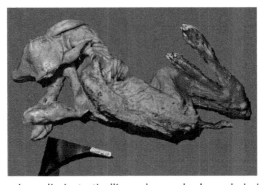

Fig. 23. Arthrogryposis, scoliosis, torticollis, and muscular hypoplasia in a newborn lamb infected in utero by Cache Valley virus.

camelids being the most susceptible. Sheep, goats, and especially cattle are relatively resistant and require large numbers of larvae for development of clinical signs, and cases are uncommon. Definitive diagnosis is by identification of the parasite in the spinal cord.

SUMMARY

This article briefly reviews some of the clinical and necropsy procedures to follow while investigating cases of neurologic disease in food animals, such as obtaining a thorough history; examining affected live animals, their herd mates, and their surroundings; performing a postmortem examination; and collecting samples. The article also describes and illustrates some of the gross pathology likely to be seen in food animals with neurologic diseases. It is emphasized that not all neurologic diseases are accompanied by abnormalities of the CNS, and that it is important to examine and sample the entire animal.

REFERENCES

1. Radostits OM, Gay CC, Blood DC, et al. Diseases of the nervous system. In: Veterinary medicine. A textbook of the diseases of cattle, sheep, pigs, goats and horses. London: W. B. Saunders; 1999. p. 501–49.
2. Constable PD. Clinical examination of the ruminant nervous system. Vet Clin North Am Food Anim Pract 2004;20:185–214.
3. Scott PR. Diagnostic techniques and clinicopathologic findings in ruminant neurologic disease. Vet Clin North Am Food Anim Pract 2004;20:215–30.
4. Stokol T, Divers TJ, Arrigan JW, et al. Cerebrospinal fluid findings in cattle with central nervous system disorders: a retrospective study of 102 cases (1990-2008). Vet Clin Pathol 2009;38:103–12.
5. D'Angelo A, Miniscalco B, Bellino C, et al. Analysis of cerebrospinal fluid from 20 calves after storage for 24 hours. Vet Rec 2009;164:491–3.
6. Andrews JJ, Van Alstine WG, Schwartz KJ. A basic approach to food animal necropsy. Vet Clin North Am Food Anim Pract 1986;2:1–29.
7. Johnson DD, Libal MC. Necropsy of sheep and goats. Vet Clin North Am Food Anim Pract 1986;2:129–46.
8. Thacker HL. Necropsy of the feeder pig and adult swine. Vet Clin North Am Food Anim Pract 1986;2:173–86.
9. Mason GL, Madden DJ. Performing the field necropsy examination. Vet Clin North Am Food Anim Pract 2007;23:503–26.
10. Nietfeld JC. Field necropsy techniques and proper specimen submission for investigation of emerging infectious diseases of food animals. Vet Clin North Am Food Anim Pract 2010;26:1–13.
11. Cornell University College of Veterinary Medicine. Virtual vet: bovine necropsy module. Available at: http://video.vet.cornell.edu/virtualvet/bovine/chapters1-4. html. Accessed January 15, 2012.
12. McCoy MA, Hutchinson T, Davidson G, et al. Postmortem biochemical markers of experimentally induced hypomagnesaemic tetany in cattle. Vet Rec 2001;148: 268–73.
13. McCoy MA. Hypomagnesaemia and new data on vitreous humor magnesium concentration as a post-mortem marker in ruminants. Magnes Res 2004;17(2): 137–45.
14. Callan RJ, Van Metre DC. Viral diseases of the ruminant nervous system. Vet Clin North Am Food Anim Pract 2004;20:327–62.

15. Centers for Disease Control and Prevention. Protocol for postmortem diagnosis of rabies in animals by direct fluorescent antibody testing. Available at: http://www.cdc.gov/rabies/pdf/rabiesdfaspv2.pdf. Accessed January 15, 2012.
16. Morin DE. Brainstem and cranial nerve abnormalities: listeriosis, otitis media/interna, and pituitary abscess syndrome. Vet Clin North Am Food Anim Pract 2004;20: 243–73.
17. Maxie MG, Youssef S. Nervous system. In: Maxie MG, editor. Jubb, Kennedy, and Palmer's pathology of domestic animals, vol. 1, 5th edition. Philadephia: Elsevier Saunders; 2007. p. 281–457.
18. Summers BA, Cummings JF, de Lahunta A. Malformations of the central nervous system. In: Veterinary neuropathology. St. Louis (MO): Mosby; 1995. p. 68–94.
19. Kupferschmidt K. New animal virus takes northern Europe by Surprise. Science Now 2012. Available at: http://news.sciencemag.org/sciencenow/2012/01/new-animal-virus-takes-northern-.html. Accessed January 20, 2012.
20. Washburn KE, Streeter RN. Congenital defects of the ruminant nervous system. Vet Clin North Am Food Anim Pract 2004;20:413–34.
21. Summers BA, Cummings JF, de Lahunta A. Degenerative diseases of the central nervous system. In: Veterinary neuropathology. St. Louis (MO): Mosby; 1995. p. 208–350.
22. Thompson K. Bones and joints. In: Maxie MG, editor. Jubb, Kennedy, and Palmer's pathology of domestic animals, vol. 1, 5th edition. Philadephia: Elsevier Saunders; 2007. p. 1–184.
23. Packer RA. Congenital and inherited anomalies of the nervous system. In: Kahn CM, editor. The Merck veterinary manual. 10th edition. Whitehouse Station (NJ): Merck & Co; 2010. p. 1118–31.

Clinical Diagnosis of Foot and Leg Lameness in Cattle

Jan K. Shearer, DVM, MS[a], Sarel R. Van Amstel, BVSc, M MED VET[b],
Bruce W. Brodersen, DVM, MS, PhD[c],*

KEYWORDS

- Bovine lameness • Cattle lameness • Lameness diagnosis • Locomotor diseases
- Record keeping

KEY POINTS

- Posture and locomotion are important observations for assessment of foot and leg health in cattle.
- A lameness evaluation should always start with a thorough examination of the foot.
- The diagnosis of foot and claw (hoof) lesions may be determined by considering the visual appearance of the lesions, foot, or claw zone affected.
- Advances in computer hardware and software have facilitated the capture of lameness and foot care information on-farm.
- Upper leg lameness presents diagnostic challenges that begin with obtaining a history of clinical signs and previous treatment, and proceeds with careful observation of posture and gait, palpation of joints, muscles, tendons and bones; manipulation of the limb to assess areas of pain, and other diagnostic procedures.

Incidence of clinical lameness exceeds that of most other diseases in many herds. Detection remains a challenge because cows are good at disguising discomfort. Evaluating posture and gait can help to identify the subtle signs of lameness so intervention can occur before the disorder has progressed. Once a cow is identified as lame, the next steps are to conduct a thorough examination to determine its source (ie, foot, claw, upper leg, or elsewhere) and apply an appropriate treatment. In many herds, it all

The authors have nothing to disclose regarding any relationship with a commercial company that has a direct financial interest in the subject matter or materials discussed in their article or with a company making a competing product.

[a] Dairy Production Medicine, Lameness, Animal Welfare, Department of Veterinary Diagnostic and Production Animal Medicine, College of Veterinary Medicine, 2436 Lloyd Vet Med Center, Iowa State University, Ames, IA 50011, USA; [b] Department of Large Animal Clinical Sciences, College of Veterinary Medicine, The University of Tennessee, 2407 River Drive, Knoxville, TN 37996, USA; [c] Veterinary Diagnostic Center, School of Veterinary Medicine and Biomedical Sciences, University of Nebraska-Lincoln, 1900 North 42nd Street, Lincoln, NE 68506-0907, USA
* Corresponding author.
E-mail address: bbrodersen1@unl.edu

ends with treatment. Contrasted to dairy cattle, in which the histories of the environment, handling, and diets of the animals are often known, feedlot cattle often come from several, often unknown, sources. In those situations, with little knowledge of prior handling, environment, and rations, feedlot personnel are often working in a black box when trying to evaluate factors involved in cases of lameness.

Owners or managers may be aware of an increase in overall herd lameness. Until they know about the occurrence of specific disorders (eg, sole ulcers, white line disease, or digital dermatitis) and rates of these conditions, it may be hard to identify underlying causes and develop a rational management strategy to address them. The collection and maintenance of records are time consuming and represent a significant cost of doing business. In the United States, compatibility with farm record-keeping systems such as the Dairy Herd Improvement Association or other systems is an important objective. This permits data on lameness to be incorporated into the farm's database on animals so that as summary reports (on individual cows or on the herd) are retrieved, other pertinent information (eg, milk production, reproductive status, etc) can be reviewed. In this article, the authors discuss the next step, which is to capture this information for better management of individual cows and herd lameness.

CLINICAL DIAGNOSIS OF FOOT LAMENESS

Most lameness in dairy cattle is associated with disorders of the foot. Observation indicates that nearly 90% of lameness involves the foot. In conditions that affect the foot, nearly 90% involve the rear feet and most (70%–90%) affect the lateral claw. Although nutrition is frequently cited as an underlying cause, the distribution of disorders to the outer claw of the rear foot suggests something different. When a cow develops laminitis, the vascular insult is not limited to the outer claw. All claws are affected. Result research indicates that lameness is complicated by metabolic factors,[1–4] such as housing and management conditions[5] that require prolonged standing on hard-flooring surfaces and natural weight-bearing forces that contribute to mechanical overloading of claws as a result of horn overgrowth.[6] Therefore, lameness occurs most commonly in the medial claw of front feet and the lateral claw of back feet. Posture and gait abnormalities may offer some suggestions regarding the cause of claw lesions. A specific diagnosis requires a careful examination of the foot.

Beyond the underlying metabolic and physical factors associated with claw disorders are infectious disorders of the foot skin and sometimes deeper tissues. These bear a close relationship to housing and environmental conditions that result in the contamination of feet with organic matter and moisture. Diagnosis of these conditions is generally made through the visual observation of lesions.

OBSERVATION FOR DETECTION OF POSTURAL ABNORMALITIES

Much can be learned from just observing an animal and its posture quietly from a distance. Cows with pain in a foot or feet will naturally attempt to reduce weight bearing in the affected foot or feet. In **Fig. 1**, a cow stands with its front legs crossed because of bilateral sole ulcers in the medial claws. Because more weight is normally borne on the medial claws, crossing the front legs will eliminate or at least reduce weight bearing on the medial claws and thus reduce some of the discomfort. A lesion in the outer claw of the front foot will cause the cow to stand with a base-wide posture of the front legs. Shifting of weight from one side to the other is also indicative of foot discomfort and may provide a clue regarding which foot is involved. Lameness is most often associated with a lesion in the outer claw in the rear legs. In these situations, the cow will stand with the foot or feet abducted or, as viewed from the rear, with feet in

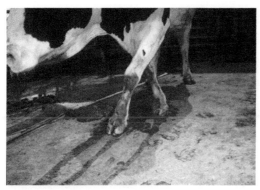

Fig. 1. Standing with front legs crossed as a consequence of bilateral sole ulcers in the medial claws.

a "cow-hocked" posture. By rotating the claws outward, the cow is able to displace more weight to the inner claws.

REAR VIEW OF HINDLIMB POSTURE (LEG SCORE SYSTEM)

This system, based on the work of Toussaint Raven,[6] is used to make a determination of a cow's or herd's need for trimming. Research has demonstrated a correlation between hindlimb posture as seen from the rear and overgrowth of the claws. In non-lame cows that are not experiencing overgrowth of the lateral claws, the back legs are straight and parallel. As the outer claw of the rear leg becomes overgrown, particularly at the heel and sole, the cow becomes progressively more cow-hocked (by rotating her feet outward) in an attempt to displace more weight on the inner claw.

Leg score is determined by the angle of the spine in relation to the interdigital space created by the outward rotation of the feet. It is graded as 1, normal (no deviation); 2, 17° to 24° deviation, and 3, greater than 24° deviation. Recommendations for the application of the leg score system are as follows: whole herd trimming is indicated if (1) less than 40% of the herd attains a score of 1, (2) more than 20% of cows attain a score of 3, or (3) more than 50% of cows attain a score of 2 or 3.

Other postural abnormalities associated with lameness include lowering of the head and arching of the spine, shoulders, and hips. Sometimes animals will lean to one side or the other, attempting to reduce weight bearing on the foot coincident with problem. A cow with laminitis will stand in a "camped under" (**Fig. 2**) posture whereby she will hold both the front and rear legs beneath her. Cows with heel lesions stand on their toes, which causes the toe to wear more and become shorter. Cows with toe lesions place more weight on the heels, which results in overgrowth and extension of the toe. Hyperextension of the fetlock joint with concomitant relaxation of the flexor tendons may occur in chronic cases. These conformational changes (long heels or long toes) of the claw horn capsule often require correction during trimming.

OBSERVATION FOR ABNORMALITIES OF GAIT

The most useful of observations for determination of lameness is gait assessment. It is necessary to know what constitutes normal gait and what to look for when trying to discern if a cow is lame. Because cows are naturally inclined to disguise discomfort early, lameness can be difficult to detect.

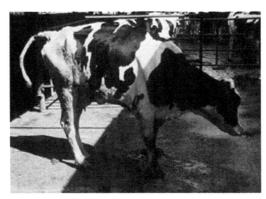

Fig. 2. Cow with acute laminitis displaying the typical "camped under" posture.

Gait characteristics are altered by conditions that make the surfaces of floors more or less slippery. On wet, manure-covered concrete floors, cows will alter their gait by slow walking speeds, changing limb angles and reducing the length of their step, in an effort to increase stability.[7–9] Hardness of the flooring surface will also affect detection of gait abnormalities. With an earthen surface traction that is more forgiving, signs of discomfort may be less exaggerated and harder to detect. Gait assessment should be performed on dry, firm flooring surface.

LOCOMOTION SCORING

Primary characteristics to assess when evaluating locomotion include walking speed (lame cows walk slower), stride length (lame cows take shorter strides), tracking (does the back foot come down where the front foot leaves the ground?), weight bearing (does the cow avoid putting weight on the leg?), posture of the spine (lame cows tend to arch their back or spine), and head bob (does the head bob up and down as the cow walks?) (**Fig. 3**).[10–12]

Locomotion scoring can be used to assess lameness in individual cows or as a tool to assess foot health on a herd basis. When used on individual cows, the purpose of lameness scoring is to identify lame cows for timely intervention, thereby limiting pain and discomfort for the cow and economic losses to the owner. Locomotion scoring on a herd basis provides a quick overview of the herd's lameness status.

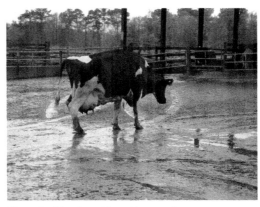

Fig. 3. Lame cow with arched back and head lowered.

One of the more prevalent locomotion scoring systems is that devised by Sprecher and colleagues,[13] which is based on the observation of spinal posture of cows while standing and walking. Although Sprecher and colleagues used the system to assess the effects of lameness on reproductive performance, in recent years the system has gained popularity as a tool for the early detection of lameness disorders in individual cows and for assessing herd foot health. Observations require that animals be observed while standing and walking on a flat surface that provides sound footing. Scores range from 1 to 5 with 1 indicating normal (ie, a cow that stands and walks with a flat back and gait is normal); 2 indicates mildly lame (ie, a cow that stands with a flat back but arches the back when walking has a normal gait); 3 indicates moderately lame (ie, a cow that has an arched back while standing and walking has a gait described as short strides in ≥1 legs); 4 indicates (ie, a cow that has an arched back while standing and walking and favors ≥1 limbs); and 5 indicates severely lame (ie, a cow has an arched back while standing and walking and refuses to place or has great difficulty placing weight on ≥1 limbs).

EXAMINATION OF THE FOOT

A thorough examination of the foot is important whether cattle are simply presented for routine preventative trimming or when observed as lame and presented for further examination and treatment. When early claw lesions are detected during the course of preventative trimming, they can be corrected at that time, preventing the possibility of the lesion progressing to a more serious condition.

Once the cow is properly restrained and the foot is secured, it should be cleaned with soap and water. Inspect the foot, particularly the interdigital skin and heel bulbs, for lesions, swelling, or evidence of foreign bodies. Focus on the claws and proceed with the 3-step functional trimming procedure described by Toussaint Raven.[6] Correction of claw horn overgrowth, early lesions, and the reestablishment of the claw capsule to its normal proportions should be part of every examination. Removal of superficial layers of horn over the white line regions of the sole and the typical site for sole ulcers helps to uncover evidence of separation, hemorrhages, or granulation tissue that might be indicative of claw lesions.

Hoof testers (**Fig. 4**) are used in cases of lameness when the lesions are not obvious. The authors' diagnostics require knowledge of whether there is pain in the claw.[14,15] The tester should be applied with firm, consistent pressure to areas where one would

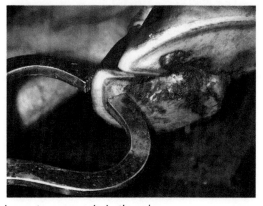

Fig. 4. Hoof tester in use to assess pain in the sole.

expect to find a lesion: the apical region of the toe, along the white line, and over the typical site for sole ulcers. It may be applied to the dorsal and abaxial wall to test for lesions underlying the wall or to detect deeper problems such as a fracture of the third phalanx (P3). It can also be used on the sole to assess sole thickness.[16,17] Extreme flexibility of the sole suggests that the sole is too thin and unlikely to support the cow's weight on a firm flooring surface such as concrete.[10,17–20]

Hoof testing can yield conflicting results as to the specific area affected (ie, foot or upper leg). Intravenous regional anesthesia can be a very useful diagnostic procedure to isolate the site of the lesion. The technique consists of placing a tourniquet above the dewclaw (**Fig. 5**) and administering approximately 20 mL of 2% lidocaine intravenously in either the medial, lateral, or dorsal digital veins. A 19-gauge butterfly catheter with a 12-inch extension tube is ideal for conducting this procedure. The needle is inserted rapidly to its hub and slowly withdrawn until the needle enters the vein and blood is flowing freely through the catheter. The lidocaine is injected slowly to avoid damage to the vein. When intravenous regional anesthesia is used for diagnostic purposes the tourniquet should be left in place for approximately 5 minutes to assure uniform distribution of the lidocaine to target tissues. The tourniquet is removed and the animal is released for gait observation. Using this technique, cows that leave the trim chute and walk away with less observable lameness are likely to have a problem in the foot. Those that show no improvement probably have a lesion in the upper leg.[14]

DIAGNOSIS BY VISUAL APPEARANCE, LOCATION, AND CLAW ZONE AFFECTED

Veterinarians and trimmers alike tend to refer to claw lesions as abscesses or sole abscesses. In fact, most are either an ulcer, white line disease, or a traumatic lesion of the sole. Foreign bodies are also common causes of traumatic sole lesions, and there are many of these, including sharp stones, wire, nails, teeth, and various other types of materials. The point is that reference to a claw lesion as an abscess or a sole abscess is useless information from a management standpoint. Knowing that the claw lesion one observes is an ulcer, white line disease, or a solar puncture, regardless of whether it has abscessed, offers the most usable information. Much

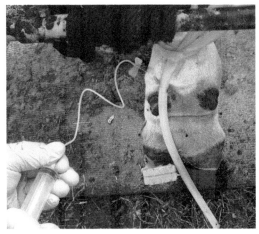

Fig. 5. Intravenous regional anesthesia using a 19-gauge butterfly catheter and 20 mL of 2% lidocaine.

of the foot work and trimming are done on farms by farm employees or foot trimmers. Some have a good understanding of proper terms and names for foot conditions and some who do not. In such cases, one may choose to rely more on the location of the lesion as identified by means of the claw zone affected.[18,21]

Foot and claw conditions are diagnosed by visual appearance, taking into consideration the location and the claw zone affected. An ulcer is defined as a full-thickness defect of the epidermis (horn) that exposes the underlying corium. Ulcers that occur in the apex of the toe (zone 5) are termed toe ulcers, those occurring at the heel–sole junction are sole ulcers (zone 4), and those occurring in the heel are heel ulcers (zone 6) (**Fig. 6**). Lesions occurring in zone 1, 2, or 3 that correspond to the areas of the white line are termed white line disease. Beyond ulcers and white line disease, one may observe traumatic lesions of the sole and/or foreign bodies in zones 1 through 6 of the weight-bearing surface. Lesions occurring in zone 0 are likely to be interdigital dermatitis, interdigital fibroma, foot rot, or digital dermatitis, and in zone 10, lesions are most often associated with digital dermatitis. If cases of heel erosion are recorded using a system such as this, they might be noted as lesions occurring in zone 6.[18]

Diagnostic details of an individual animal's lameness disorder are useful for the proper management of its specific condition; the database necessary for effective problem solving on a herd basis often requires little more than a simple enumeration of these events to be meaningful. Large herds tend to be less interested in detailed information on individuals and more interested in summary statistics that might signal errors in the areas of cow comfort, feeding, and management. Specific lesion details (ie, severity, chronicity, size, etc) regarding a toe lesion in zone 5 may offer ideas for treatment, time to recheck, a prognosis, or possible need for culling of an animal. No matter how detailed this information is, it does not offer much in answering the question of the predominant cause of lameness for a particular herd. Knowing, for example, that 20% of the last 150 cows presented to the trimmer for treatment in the past 100 days had a lesion in zone 5 provides valuable information as to a possible cause and where one might want to focus more attention for greater definition of the problem. Consider the following data set from a large dairy in South Georgia where record keeping relies almost exclusively on identification of the claw zone affected by a group of well-trained on-farm trimmers.

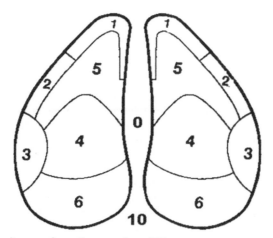

Fig. 6. Claw zone diagram from Greenough and Weaver.

Lameness was studied in a large dairy in the southeastern United States.[22] Data collected included records for 4915 cows, of which 1861 had at least one recorded lameness event:

- 20% were thin-sole toe ulcers recorded as lesions occurring in zones 1 and 2 as a result of a separation of the sole from the white line
- 16% were sole ulcers in zone 4
- 13% were thin soles, which includes zones 1 through 6
- 10% were caused by white line disease in zone 3
- 8% were heel ulcers in zone 6
- 6% were leg injuries
- 4% were injuries that caused upper leg lameness
- 2% were toe ulcers associated with laminitis and rotation of P3 in zone 5
- 20% were other conditions including digital dermatitis, corkscrew claw, and foot rot

Annual incidence risk for lameness was determined to be 49.1% and lameness rates for all lesions were highest during the summer months. In addition to these descriptive statistics for this herd, researchers were able to determine that as parity increased, so did incidence rates for thin soles, sole ulcers, white line disease, heel ulcers, and injuries. Heel, sole, and toe ulcers all occurred with greater frequency during mid-lactation. Analysis of these data clearly demonstrated that the lameness problem experienced in this herd was primarily the result of thin soles and thin-sole toe ulcers, which accounted for 33% of recorded lesions. Thin soles also predispose to thin-sole toe ulcers and a higher incidence of sole ulcers, white line disease, and heel ulcers. The recommendation to this dairy based on these data was to apply rubber flooring to travel lanes, holding areas, and eventually barns as needed to reduce the rate of claw horn wear.

PROBLEMS WITH INFORMATION ON LAMENESS IN DAIRY RECORDS

The greatest deficiency in the recording of health information has been in the area of foot care. This is especially interesting as lameness has been cited as the single most costly clinical disease of dairy cattle. Only in recent time have record-keeping systems such as Dairy Comp 305 and Dairy Herd Improvement Association records started to work on better ways to capture lameness information. It is important to point out that the deficiency is not the result of a failure of trimmers to collect the information. The problem lies with the inability to efficiently transfer this information to herd records, where it can be analyzed and interpreted.[21]

A second problem with lameness data is that they lack uniformity. Trimmers throughout the country use different terms in their descriptions of foot conditions. In some cases, the problem is related to language barriers; in others, the person collecting the information is unfamiliar with the proper terms for the various lameness conditions. Some dairymen do not understand the information even if proper terms are used. They need help interpreting the information to make necessary management changes. As described previously, all too frequently, claw conditions such as ulcers and white line disease are collectively referred to as sole abscesses or laminitis. So, the information may be available, it may be difficult to interpret because the terms used are not specific, or, in the worst case scenario, the information may be erroneous or unknown.[21]

If record keeping of lameness disorders is to become a routine management practice on dairy farms, the mechanism for collection of the information must be simple, convenient, and sufficiently comprehensive to yield information of value in decision making. This information will be of greatest interest to those who are managing lameness conditions in individual cows. For others, information on lameness disorders will be of more value as a herd monitoring and management tool. There are newer technologies that combine software and specific computer hardware with the capability for accomplishing the needs of both. It is beyond the scope of this article to completely describe these technologies.

The original concept of recording lesions by means of the use of claw zones was introduced by Greenough and Weaver in 1992. The American Association of Bovine Practitioners offered a reporting scheme that incorporated the use of a lesion code along with claw zone to record lameness conditions in 2004.[23] There did not seem to be widespread use of this reporting scheme, in part because most trimming and foot care is conducted by trimmers and not by veterinarians. A study by Cramer and colleagues,[24] in 2008, demonstrated almost perfect agreement among trimmers who were taught to use a modified version of this record-keeping system. These results were corroborated by observations from the study described earlier of the thin-sole herd in the southeastern United States. Commercial applications of this system using computer touch-screen technology have been developed in the United States (Hoof Supervisor, Supervisor Systems, Wisconsin). Additionally, a system developed in Austria by Dr Johann Kofler and colleagues uses a similar system to record and analyze foot lesion data.[25] Hoof Supervisor has gained widespread acceptance in North America (S. Martin, personal communication, 2011).

THE ALBERTA DAIRY HOOF HEALTH PROJECT AND HOOF SUPERVISOR

Beyond the need for information to better understand lameness in individual herds is the need to understand lameness from a regional, state, province, and national perspective. This affords the opportunity for herd-to-herd, region-to-region, etc, comparisons. The best example of this is the Alberta Dairy Hoof Health Project (S. Martin, personal communication, 2011). As of August 20, 2011, 147 Alberta herds and 69 herds from British Columbia had contributed trimming records and DHI data to The Alberta Dairy Hoof Health Project's hoof health database, including records for 35,229 individual cows. In Alberta, 48.6% of these cows had one or more of the 14 claw lesions documented by hoof trimmers in this project; in British Columbia, 57.5% of cows trimmed had one or more of these lesions. The top 5 of these lesions from the Alberta Hoof Health Project are listed in **Table 1**.

Table 1
Summary data on selected conditions from the Alberta Dairy Hoof Health Project

	Alberta		British Columbia	
Participating farms	147		69	
Total distinct cows	27,092		8137	
Cows with lesions	13,174	48.6%	4679	57.5%
Digital dermatitis	8164	44.9%	2581	40.3%
Sole ulcer	2999	16.5%	821	12.8%
White line lesion	2559	14.1%	846	13.2%
Sole hemorrhage	1103	6.1%	490	7.6%
Toe ulcer	888	4.9%	335	5.2%

Preliminary results point to a high prevalence of digital dermatitis and claw horn disruption (S. Martin, personal communication, 2011).

Digital dermatitis was by far the most common lesion observed, accounting for 48% of all lesions recorded. Next in order of decreasing prevalence were sole ulcer, white line lesion, sole hemorrhage, and toe ulcer. Combined, these 4 lesions accounted for 41.8% of all lesions recorded. All data were collected by trimmers using Hoof Supervisor, which forwards the information from the herds to a central source for summarization of the data from both provinces. The long-term objectives of this project are to determine the most common causes of lameness and the specific areas of hoof health that need further research (S. Martin, personal communication, 2011).

SPECIFIC DISORDERS OF FEET
Deep Digital Sepsis Conditions

There are at least 3 clinical entities that may be observed: (1) avulsion of the deep digital flexor tendon and retroarticular space abscess formation, (2) infection of the distal interphalangeal joint (DIP), and (3) heel abscess (**Fig. 7**).[10–12,14,26]

Avulsion of the deep digital flexor tendon occurs after osteitis and a pathologic fracture of the flexor tuberosity of P3. This is most commonly observed as a secondary complication of a chronic sole ulcer. The lesion begins as an ascending infection that extends upward through the corium and digital cushion and into the flexor tuberosity of P3.[10,11,14,26] Other structures that may be involved include the navicular bursa, deep flexor tendon sheath, and surrounding tissues. Abscess formation in the retroarticular space located between the second phalanx and the deep flexor tendon is a common sequela. These changes often occur without involvement of the DIP.

Infection of the DIP occurs via 3 primary routes: an ascending infection through the sole or white line may extend to the joint either (1) proximal to the navicular bone via the palmar/plantar pouch of the DIP joint that is located adjacent to the retroarticular space; (2) via breakdown of the ligamentous attachment between the ligamentous

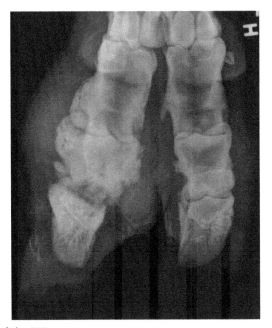

Fig. 7. Infection of the DIP.

attachment of the distal part of the navicular bone and P3, or (3) via the extension of infection from the interdigital skin (foot rot) through the axial joint capsule or dorsal pouch of the DIP joint capsule.[10,11,14,26]

Heel abscesses occur most commonly via the extension of a white line disease abscess (zone 3) or a heel abscess (zone 6). These are often simple to treat as they often localize in the fibroelastic pad of the heel retinaculum.

Diagnosis of Deep Digital Sepsis Conditions

Foot rot usually presents as a generalized swelling of the foot that extends to or above the dew claws. In most cases, this swelling is accompanied by a painful necrotic lesion in the interdigital skin and severe lameness. Although the conditions just described may be similar in appearance, they are often unilateral in their occurrence. Careful examination is important for determination of the most likely underlying cause.

Start by cleaning the foot and interdigital skin with soap, water, and a brush. Examine the foot, claws, interdigital area, and heel bulbs for areas of swelling, injury, or other abnormality. Assuming all is normal, using a hoof knife, or preferably an angle grinder with a coarse grinding disk, clean the soles of each claw by removal of a superficial layer of horn that will permit examination of the white line for evidence of separation. Also, examine the skin horn junction both axially and abaxially for evidence of loose horn. If such areas are found, use the hook of the hoof knife to explore the extent to which the horn is undermined. Remove all loose horn until reaching the point at which the horn is reattached to the underlying corium.

In the case of retroarticular space abscesses, it is not uncommon to find a chronic sole ulcer adjacent to the swollen heel (**Fig. 8**). In most cases, one can find a draining tract that with pressure on the heel will exude purulent material. This tract should be gently probed with a teat cannula or other probing device to determine the extent and location of the abscess capsule. Once the probe is inserted to the full extent of the tract/abscess, it can be left in place to serve as a guide for surgical correction of the problem. Gentle probing of draining purulent tracts is a useful diagnostic procedure for determination of the primary location of abscess capsules. In most cases, there will be evidence of avulsion of the deep flexor tendon, which causes the toe of the affected claw to rotate upward.

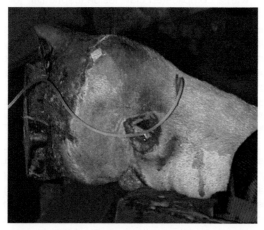

Fig. 8. Retroarticular space abscess. Intravenous regional anesthesia is being applied for surgical correction.

Septic arthritis of the DIP is characterized by a prominent swelling of the coronet that extends upward to the fetlock. This condition is sometimes accompanied by a discharging tract on the craniolateral aspect of the coronet that is considered by many to be near pathognomic for septic arthritis of the distal interphalangeal joint. As with retroarticular space abscesses, animals with septic DIP joints exhibit severe lameness that is difficult to alleviate even with a foot block applied to the healthy unaffected claw.[10,11,14,26]

Fractures of the Claw Capsule and P3

Traumatic fractures of the claw capsule are not uncommon and may occur in a multitude of ways. Sometimes they are accompanied by fracture of P3. These may be caused by slatted flooring in trailers and barns, rails or side boards in a gate or fence, or other structural obstruction that results in the claw becoming wedged or stuck and subsequently dislodged by a rapid twisting, sideward, or other movement of the foot and lower leg. Extent of the damage and corrective measures begin with intravenous regional anesthesia and close inspection of the claw for fractures of P3 that may require removal of the fractured portion of the bone and other permanently damaged tissues.

Traumatically induced fractures of P3 may also occur without visible evidence of trauma to the claw horn capsule. Animals that exhibit severe pain in a claw but with no indication of white line disease, puncture of the sole, or other lesion present a significant diagnostic challenge that often requires a radiograph for confirmation of the fracture. Diagnostic anesthesia of the foot to determine if pain is in fact coming primarily from the foot or upper leg is also useful.

Another cause of fracture of the P3 that may not be accompanied by external evidence on the claw capsule is that related to pathophysiologic factors. These are sometimes detected radiographically or they may be found during the process of corrective trimming of toe lesions. Removal of necrotic foul-smelling horn and purulent material in the toe of the claw sometimes leads to the isolation of a sequestrum that is actually the apex of P3. Often, removal of the sequestrum and associated necrotic tissue is sufficient to provide long-term relief.[10,11,14]

Septic Tenosynovitis

Swelling associated with a complicated claw lesion (septic DIP joint or retroarticular space abscess) that extends well above the fetlock is highly suggestive of septic tenosynovitis. Diagnosis may be confirmed by aspirating fluid from the sheath with a needle and syringe. Sepsis of the tendon and tendon sheath is indicated by a total white cell count of more than 25,000/μL and a total protein of more than 4.5 g/dL. Ultrasonography of the tendons that demonstrates the presence of floating echogenic particles in the compartments of the flexor tendon sheath may also be used to confirm tenosynovitis. A 7.5-MHz probe is preferred by these authors for making this assessment.[10,14]

Injuries/Conditions Involving Loss of the Claw Capsule (Also Known as "Degloving" Injuries)

Degloving-type lesions most often occur as a consequence of injuries whereby an animal's foot may become stuck or wedged between 2 objects and, when finally removed, results in loss of the claw horn capsule. These are diagnosed by simple observation that demonstrates complete or partial loss of the horn shell. These usually involve 1 claw, but on occasion both claws may be involved. Although these lesions may seem catastrophic, depending on the severity of the damage to the underlying corium tissues, most will heal uneventfully if the animal is offered appropriate care.[11]

Emphasis in managing these conditions is to clean the lesions and remove loose horn or any foreign material that may be lodged in or impinging on the exposed corium tissues. If only 1 claw is affected, apply a foot block to the healthy unaffected claw to relieve weight bearing on the damaged claw. Application of a nonirritating topical medication beneath a loose bandage should be applied to protect delicate corium tissues. If both claws are affected, the animal should be restricted from movement on hard flooring surfaces and housed in a well-bedded area.

Laminitis

Laminitis manifests as clinical disease with rapid onset of acute pain and lameness (see **Fig. 2**). This occurs as the result of metabolic acidosis shortly after alimentary overload of readily fermentable carbohydrates. With carbohydrate overload, there is systemic release of vasoactive substances that reduce blood flow in the hoof and thus an interruption in production of hoof wall and sole by germinal epithelial cells.[27] Clinical signs of lameness can be seen as soon as 24 to 33 hours after carbohydrate overload.[28] Histologic lesions of laminitis can be detected as soon as 48 hours after carbohydrate overload. Laminitis can have differing degrees of severity. The most severely affected cases are manifested by breakdown of the suspensory tissue that holds P3 suspended in the hoof. This breakdown leads to separation of the hoof wall from the corium and rotation of the P3 in the hoof. After separation of the corium from the hoof wall, there is abnormal hoof growth resulting in the classic presentation of overgrown hooves that curl upward. In cases of laminitis, there can be interruption in production of hoof wall and sole by germinal epithelial cells. This is manifested by the presence of horizontal bands in the hoof wall and, in some cases, clefts in the sole (**Fig. 9**).

Papillomatous Digital Dermatitis (Hairy Heel Warts)

Papillomatous digital dermatitis (PPD) has been long recognized as a cause of lameness in cattle.[29] Beginning as a mild superficial dermatitis, PPD progresses to a proliferative and erosive lesion (**Fig. 10**). This lesion is characterized by marked dermal thickening, as a result of proliferation of granulation tissue, marked hyperkeratosis, and growth of papillomatous projections of epidermis.[30] These proliferative lesions are heavily colonized by spirochetes that extend into the stratum spinosum. Previously, *Treponema phagedenis*–like spirochetes were isolated from cases of PPD,[31] and recently, PPD has been experimentally reproduced by cultures of mixed

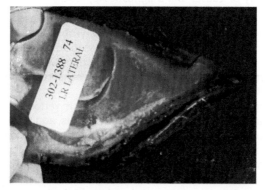

Fig. 9. Cleft in sole as a result of prior episode of laminitis. Note separation of distal phalanx from hoof wall (*arrow*). (*Courtesy of* Bruce Brodersen, DVM, PhD, Lincoln, NE.)

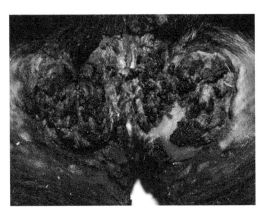

Fig. 10. Heel of feedlot steer with papillomatous digital dermatitis. (*Courtesy of* Alan R. Doster, DVM, PhD, Lincoln, NE.)

treponemes grown from tissues derived from natural cases of PPD.[32] Treatment has been successful with topical application of various antibiotics.[33]

SPECIFIC DISORDERS OF LEGS
Approach to Diagnosis of Upper Leg Lameness in Cattle

When dealing with upper leg lameness, the first step is to obtain a history in terms of the duration, severity, onset of clinical signs, and any previous treatment. This information is useful for making a reasonable prognosis and for deciding on possible follow-up treatment approaches.

Examination begins with an observation of the animal from a distance while standing and walking. This is followed by hands-on examination techniques that, for the upper leg, include palpation during standing and walking and manipulation of the leg with the animal in lateral recumbency (ie, lying on its side). In some cases, it may be difficult to distinguish upper from lower leg problems. As described previously, this can be done by placing a tourniquet at the level of the fetlock joint followed by intravenous injection of 20 mL of 2% lidocaine into a vein below the tourniquet. Remove the tourniquet after 5 minutes or so and immediately allow the animal to walk. In cases of upper leg problems, the lameness will persist.[19]

Front Legs (Summary of Causes and Diagnostic Approach)

Inability to advance or difficulty in advancing the leg may be associated with supra-scapular or radial nerve injury or bicipital bursitis (**Table 2**).[34] In addition, the leg may be held in semiflexion with the elbow dropped in the case of damage to the radial nerve at the level of the brachial plexus.[10] The radial nerve innervates the extensor muscles of the carpus and foot and serves to provide sensory innervation to the lateral skin of the forelimb from the elbow to the carpus.[35]

Lesions involving the eighth cervical and first thoracic vertebrae result in paralysis that prevents an animal from extending its elbow, carpus, and fetlock to bear weight. The elbow is dropped, the carpus and fetlock are in partial flexion, and the limb is dragged, causing abrasion to the dorsal surface of the foot.[35] In the absence of fractures and obvious muscle damage, difficulty advancing the limb and an inability to extend the elbow, carpus, and fetlock to bear weight, in combination with an absence of skin sensation on the lateral and dorsal surface of the lower limb, confirm radial nerve paralysis.[36]

Table 2	
Common causes and diagnostic approach for front upper leg lameness	
Cause	**Diagnostic Clinical Signs and Procedures**
Suprascapular nerve	Atrophy of supraspinatus and infraspinatus Inability to extend shoulder and abduct the limb Lower limb reflexes Sensation intact
Proximal radial nerve	Elbow: dropped Inability to extend elbow and lower leg and advanced the leg Leg in flexed position/loss of skin sensation lateral and dorsal on lower limb
Distal radial nerve	Elbow: normal position Inability to extend lower leg/leg in flexed position Loss of skin sensation lateral and dorsal on lower limb
Bicipital bursitis	Decrease flexion of elbow Shortened stride/increased fluid in bursa on ultrasound

Carpal and fetlock
  flexor deformity
  (contracted tendons)
	Walks on toes and knuckles forward
	Walks on dorsum of foot
	Unable to straighten the leg or bear weight
	Unable to rise
	Superficial and deep flexor contracture/tendons of flexor carpi
	  radialis and ulnaris tight on palpation

Septic arthritis	Joint swollen, hot, painful Joint effusion on palpation, ultrasound Joint fluid has high white blood cell count and protein Predominant neutrophil population Degenerate/bacteria sometimes

Clinical signs of suprascapular nerve injury include stumbling, inability to support weight in severe cases, inability to support and extend the shoulder, a shorten stride, and abduction of the leg. Reflexes and sensation in the lower limb remain normal if only the nerve is affected. Atrophy of the supraspinatus and infraspinatus muscles may become visible as early as 5 to 7 days post injury.[34] With bicipital bursitis, the brachial biceps muscle and its bursa can be visualized ultrasonographically in a transverse plane in the cranial shoulder region. In cases of bursitis, there is an increase in the amount of fluid in the bursa.[37]

In calves, contracture of the flexors (ie, clinically referred to as "contracted tendons") may cause flexion of both the carpus and fetlock.[38] In such cases, the leg usually cannot be straightened, and the flexor carpi ulnaris and flexor carpi radialis can be felt as tight bands at the back of the knee in addition to the superficial and deep digital flexors.[38] Semiflexion of the knee can also be caused by abnormal conformation or metabolic bone disease. Depending on the level of contracture of the flexors, only the fetlock may be in various degrees of flexion. In milder cases, the animal may be able to walk on its toes and knuckle forward during weight bearing. In more severe cases, the animal bears weight on the dorsum of the foot.[38] The superficial and deep flexor tendons and the suspensory ligament of the proximal sesamoid feel tight on palpation.[38]

The carpus is one of the common joints affected in cases of septic arthritis in calves.[37] The joint is warm and often painful, and there is a palpable effusion in the joint. Use of ultrasound over the longitudinal plane of the dorsal surface of the joint will facilitate arthrocentesis. Individual joint recesses that can be visualized include the radiocarpal, intercarpal, and carpometacarpal joints. In the absence of ultrasound, joint fluid can usually be obtained from the radiocarpal pouch with the carpus in slight flexion.[37] A high white cell count in the presence of degenerate neutrophils confirms septic arthritis. Bacteria may not always be visible on the slide. In chronic cases, the joint looks and feels thicker and has reduced range of motion. In such cases, chronic degenerative changes will be visible radiographically,[39] and may be initially detected over the cranial surfaces of the proximal carpal row. The radiocarpal joint space will be widened, and subchondral bone destruction along with new bone formation may be observed simultaneously.[39]

Back Legs (Summary of Causes and Diagnostic Approach)

Knuckling at the fetlock may indicate lesions of the spine, sciatic, peroneal, or tibial nerves; dropping of the hock during standing but more so during walking often indicates gastrocnemius rupture; overextension of the hock is associated with peroneal nerve damage, peroneus tersius rupture, upper fixation of the patella, flexor tendon contracture, straight hocks (post hocks), and advanced degenerative joint disease[10,39]; intermittent spastic contracture of both legs with flexion of the hock is caused by spasmodic syndrome, whereas spastic contracture of one or both hind legs with overextension of the hock is caused by spastic paresis[40]; and asymmetry of the pelvis may be caused by hip dislocation or other lesions involving the pelvis (**Table 3**).

Table 3	
Common causes and diagnostic approach for back upper leg lameness	
Cause	**Diagnostic Clinical Signs and Procedures**
Hip joint dislocation–dorsal	Cow up or down/asymmetry in hips Crepitation over hip area/leg shorter and hock higher than opposite leg Radiographs
Hip dislocation–caudoventral	Cow down Femoral head in obturator foramen Radiographs
Anterior cruciate rupture	Increased laxity in stifle Audible noise during movement Joint effusion
Medial collateral ligament rupture	Increased joint space medially Instability of medial meniscus
Upward patella fixation	Limb locked in extension Exaggerated motion during flexion
Peroneus tersius rupture	Overextended hock Tibia and metatarsus can be extended to 180° Swelling cranial on tibia
Peroneal neuropathy	Overextended hock Knuckling of fetlock Decreased skin sensation on dorsal surface of metatarsus and fetlock
Tibial neuropathy	Dropped hock Knuckling of fetlock Loss of skin sensation palmar aspect of lower limb
Partial sciatic neuropathy	Bilateral dropped hocks Knuckling of fetlocks

Instability within the stifle joint associated with cranial cruciate rupture is often seen when the animal is walking and may be accompanied by an audible sound (click). This is caused by sliding of the femoral condyles over the tibial plateau.[39] The animal tends to stand with the fetlock slightly flexed and the heel raised. Weight bearing is primarily on the tip of the toe. In cases of medial collateral ligament instability, the leg is held in an abducted position to relieve weight bearing on the medial side of the stifle and weight is placed on the medial claw when walking.[39] Upward fixation of the patella will cause the limb to "lock" when in full extension, resulting in a stringhalt-type exaggerated motion during flexion. The animal may have a normal gait in between steps. Rarely, the leg may become locked in extension.[10,39]

With superficial flexor tendon contracture, the proximal interphalangeal joint may become subluxated, resulting in knuckling of the joint.[38] The animal may walk and stand on its toe and the leg may seem to be shorter than the opposite side. With gastrocnemius rupture, the hock is dropped and partially flexed and moves farther down when walking. The fetlock may knuckle during locomotion.[10] Tibial nerve paralysis also results in a dropped hock and slight knuckling of the fetlock. The hock remains dropped while the animal is walking but does not sink during weight bearing compared with rupture of the gastrocnemius muscle.[10]

Obturator nerve paralysis primarily affects the adductor muscles of the inner thigh of the rear legs. Affected animals have a wide base stance and may seem ataxic, and they are predisposed to splaying their back legs.[10] Cows with damage to the peroneal nerve will stand with the foot knuckled over onto the dorsum of the pastern and fetlock joint. At the same time, the hock joint will seem to be overextended. In mild cases, the fetlock tends to knuckle over intermittently when the cow walks.[10] General indicators of an upper leg lameness problem include joint or soft tissue swelling.

DISORDERS INVOLVING SPECIFIC JOINTS OF THE REAR LEG
Hip Joint

Slight abduction of the back leg with outward rotation of the toe is often associated with lesions in the stifle or hip.[39] Crepitation (crackling or grating) may be felt while rocking the animal sideways with one or both hands on the greater trochanter. Crepitation, however, is not a reliable sign of the presence of lesions within the hip joint.[39] What sometimes feels like crepitation may turn out to be a normal joint, and crepitation originating from the stifle may be interpreted as coming from the hip.

Specific problems may include rupture of the round ligament in the hip joint, hip dislocation; pelvic fractures; fractures of the head of the femur, slipped capital femoral epiphysis, or severe coxitis.[39] The relative position of the greater trochanter to the tuber coxae and the tuber ischia should be determined and should form a triangle with the ventral point representing the greater trochanter t.[41] This triangle is lost with craniodorsal luxation with the greater trochanter being placed in-line with the tuber coxae and tuber ischia.[41] With caudoventral dislocation, the trochanter major may not be palpable.[41] A rectal examination should be performed to determine the presence of crepitation while moving the animal from side to side or of hard bony protrusions, which may indicate the presence of a pelvic fracture.

More frequently, the animal will be down particularly with fractures or caudoventral hip dislocation. Examination should be carried out with the animal in lateral recumbency. With craniodorsal displacement, the leg may seem shortened and the hock higher than the opposite hock.[39] Abduction and adduction and rotation of the leg by an assistant while both hands of the examiner are cupped over the greater trochanter may elicit crepitation. Manipulation is more painful with caudoventral dislocation and the animal resists flexion of the leg. It is possible to palpate the femoral head in the obturator foramen in the case of caudoventral dislocation.[39]

Ultrasound-guided arthrocentesis can be carried out in cases in which an increase in joint fluid can be visualized. Ultrasound is carried out in a longitudinal-oblique plane with the transducer placed parallel to the long axis of the femoral neck and moving it craniodorsally to where a line drawn between the 2 tuber coxae intersects the longitudinal axis of the vertebral column.[37] Radiographs are useful in establishing the cause of the lameness. The animal should be anesthetized and placed in dorsal recumbency. The size of the musculature will to a large extent determine the detail visible in the radiograph.[39]

Stifle Joint

Severity of lameness can vary depending on structures involved such as the cranial cruciate ligament, menisci, or the collateral ligaments in addition to the time after onset of the problem. Examination in the standing animal involves palpation of the joint for fluid effusion and stability. Demonstration of instability of the joint can be done in the following ways: the examiner stands behind the animal and reach around the leg with both hands. Lock the fingers over the tibial crest while leaning into the back of the thigh. The leg is stabilized against that of the examiner while the tibia is pulled back. Alternatively, the examiner may stand in front of the affected leg and try to demonstrate laxity by pushing on the tibial crest.[41] The foot has to be stabilized during this procedure. Distention of the joint capsule can cause swelling between the patellar ligaments despite the presence of the fat pad. In addition, there are extensions of the joint capsule between the quadriceps femoris muscle and the femur and distally around the tendons of the peroneus tertius and the long digital extensor muscle.[39,41]

To distinguish between trauma and sepsis of the joint, arthrocentesis is a useful diagnostic tool. Total cell count in nonseptic cases is normally less than 1000 cells/mL, and the polymorphonuclear cells are less than 10% of the total.[39] The following should be considered with arthrocentesis of the stifle. There is communication between the femoropatellar and medial femorotibial joint cavities. These compartments do not always communicate with the lateral femerotibial space. To enter this compartment, a needle is introduced behind the lateral patellar ligament and directed caudally. To enter the femeropatellar and the femorotibial compartments, the needle is inserted between the medial and middle patellar ligaments and directed slightly downward and toward the medial lip of the trochlea.[39,41] Use of ultrasound will confirm the presence of increased joint fluid and facilitate collection.[37]

With medial collateral ligament damage, the medial meniscus becomes detached and the joint capsule stretched, resulting in more laxity on the medial side of the joint. The limb is usually kept in an abducted position and more weight is placed on the medial claw. If the leg is pulled outward, an increase in the joint space on the medial side can be palpated and excessive movement of the medial meniscus can be demonstrated by palpation between the medial collateral ligament and the medial patellar ligament.[37]

Overly straight hocks may lead to degenerative joint disease in the stifle, resulting in lameness. There may be some joint enlargement and crepitation on movement of the joint. Radiographic changes in chronic cases will confirm the presence of chronic degenerative changes such as thickening of the joint capsule, epiphyseal deformity, and osteophyte formation at the joint margins.[37]

Lateral luxation of the patella may follow femoral nerve injury or could be congenital. Femoral nerve injury may occur after forced traction during birth. The calf is unable to support weight on the leg and the hock and stifle are flexed while walking. The patella may be luxated or can easily be moved out of the groove. Progressive atrophy of the quadriceps occurs, which gives the leg a hollowed-out appearance over the lower femur.[15,37] With upward fixation of the patella, it is important to understand that palpation of the stifle may not reveal any obvious abnormalities.[10] However, the medial patellar ligament may feel abnormally tight.

Diagnostic radiographs of the stifle can be difficult to obtain in adult cattle because of the thickness of the structures that need to be penetrated. The anteroposterior view is unrewarding. Positioning of the cassette in standing animal may be difficult, and for that reason lateral recumbency with the leg in extension may be a better choice.[39]

Hock Joint

Rupture of the peroneus muscle results in overextension of the hock because this muscle group is the primary flexors of this joint. In cattle, rupture occasionally occurs in the mid belly or at the junction of the proximal or distal tendon. If the limb is manually lifted and extended caudally, the tibia and metatarsus are in a straight line while the stifle joint remains at 90°. Damage usually results in a painful swelling over the cranial shaft of the tibia.[10]

Peroneal neuropathy may result in loss of skin sensation on the dorsal aspect of the lower limb and overextension of the leg. The peroneal nerve passes superficially over the lateral aspect of the rear leg where it is vulnerable to external trauma. It is often damaged in cows that suffer milk fever or downer cow syndrome as a result of the cow's body weight that puts pressure on the nerve where it crosses over the bone. The hock joint will seem to be overextended in cows with damage to this nerve. In mild cases, the fetlock tends to knuckle over intermittently when the cow walks.[10] In severe cases, cows will experience a decreased sensation on the dorsal aspect of the fetlock. The prognosis for cows affected with peroneal nerve damage depends on the severity of the nerve injury. Recovery may take days to months depending on severity.[10,36]

Overflexion of the hock is seen with gastrocnemius rupture. There is swelling at site of rupture. The gastrocnemius muscle originates from caudal femoral surface and inserts on point of hock. Rupture can occur in 3 places: in the muscle belly, the muscle–tendon junction, which is the most common site to rupture or the insertion of the tendon on the tuber calcis. Diagnosis is based on the typical clinical signs, tendon laxity, and swelling with edema at the rupture site.[10] Differentials may include calcanean bursitis, luxation of superficial flexor tendon, or tarsal fracture. With complete rupture, the animal is down and unable to rise. The ability to fold the affected leg completely on itself is diagnostic for complete rupture.[15]

The tibial nerve innervates the palmar/plantar aspect of the skin of the lower limb, which may show partial or complete loss of sensation in cases of tibial neuropathy. Partial sciatic nerve injury following calving or trauma to the spine is usually bilateral. The cow walks with short stilted steps while both the hocks and fetlocks remain in semiflexion. The spine should be palpated and a rectal examination performed to investigate the possibility of a fracture.

Swelling of the hock joint is usually associated with peritarsal bursitis, septic arthritis of the hock joint, or swelling caused by degenerative joint disease, which may or may not be associated with post hocks.[10,39] Peritarsal bursitis is a chronic cellulitis involving the lateral aspect of the hock joints. It is usually bilateral. Lameness is usually absent except in cases that cause mechanical impairment of the joint or in cases of severe abscessation or septic arthritis. In such cases, the animal may become severely lame with a discharging tract over the lateral aspect of the joint. The swollen joint may feel warm, fluctuant, and painful to touch or manipulation. Needle aspirate will confirm the presence of an exudate.

A peritarsal abscess should be distinguished from a septic joint. This can be done with the use of ultrasound. The tibiotarsal pouch communicates with the proximal intertarsal compartment but not the distal intertarsal and tarsometatarsal compartments. An abscess will show as a walled-off cavity outside the joint filled with fluid with a cellular appearance.[37]

In cases of chronic degenerative joint disease, the joint swelling will be hard and less painful compared with acute or subacute septic tarsitis. The needle is inserted on the dorsal surface medial to the extensor tendons and at the level of articulation between the tibia and proximal tarsal bones.[10] Degenerative changes within the joint may also be associated with chronic infections such as those caused by *Mycoplasma* sp. Chronic bone changes within the joint can be shown radiographically.

Fetlock Joint

Instability (flexion during weight bearing or knuckling) of the fetlock can result from spinal injury caused by trauma such as getting caught under the sides of the free stall or spinal lymphosarcoma. Damage to the sciatic nerve (particularly the peroneal branch of the sciatic) will result in knuckling of the fetlock joint. Conditions of the back of the foot such as sole ulcer or severe digital dermatitis may also cause knuckling as a result of redistribution of weight toward the toe.[41] The foot should always be examined for the presence of lesions that may cause the animal to knuckle.

Peroneal nerve paralysis is a common secondary complication with milk fever, downer cow syndrome, or other conditions that may cause a cow to remain down for an extended period of time. In severe cases, cows will experience a decreased sensation on the dorsal surface of the fetlock. Overextension of the fetlock may occur following flexor tendon rupture or rupture of the suspensory ligaments of the proximal sesamoid. The fetlock is overextended to the point that the animal bears weight on the plantar/palmar aspect of the foot. There may be a visible swelling above the dew claws, and the presence of an effusion in the tendon sheath or core lesions in the flexor tendons may be visible on ultrasound.[37]

SUMMARY

The causes of lameness in cattle are multifactorial and involve a combination of housing, management, and environmental factors and a variety of infectious agents. There can be white line disease with white line separation, laminitis, and ascending infection into the hoof, leading to tenosynovitis. Arriving at a cause can often require concerted efforts during an extended period of time. A diagnosis of lameness is often based mainly on clinical observations. A detailed record of those observations over time and among several animals within a herd can provide valuable information toward solving lameness problems. Advances in computer hardware and software help facilitate more detailed collection of data and analysis of that data.

REFERENCES

1. Bicalho RC, Machado VS, Caixeta LS. Lameness in dairy cattle: a debilitating disease or a disease of debilitated cattle? A cross-sectional study of lameness prevalence and thickness of the digital cushion. J Dairy Sci 2009;92:3175–84.
2. Tarleton JF, Webster AJ. A biochemical and biomechanical basis for the pathogenesis of claw horn lesions. Proc of the 12th Int Sym on Lameness in Ruminants. Orlando (FL): 2002. p. 395–8.

3. Tarleton JF, Holah DE, Evans KM, et al. Biomechanical and histopathological changes in the support structures of bovine hooves around the time of first calving. Vet J 2002;163:196–204.

4. Webster J. Effect of environment and management on the development of claw and leg diseases. Proc of the XXII World Buiatrics Congress (keynote lectures). Hanover (Germany): 2002. p. 248–56.

5. Knott L, Tarlton JF, Craft H, et al. Effects of housing, parturition and diet change on the biochemistry and biomechanics of the support structures of the hoof of dairy heifers. Vet J 2006;174:277–87.

6. Toussaint Raven E. Cattle footcare and claw trimming. Ipswich (United Kingdom): Farming Press, Ltd; 1989.

7. Shearer JK, van Amstel SR. Effect of flooring and/or flooring surfaces on lameness disorders in dairy cattle. Proceedings of the Western Dairy Management Conference. Reno (NV), March 7–9, 2007. p. 149–159.

8. Somers JG, Schouten WG, Frankena K, et al. Development of claw traits and claw lesions in dairy cows kept on different floor systems. J Dairy Sci 2005;88: 110–20.

9. Vanegas J, Overton M, Berry SL, et al. Effect of rubber flooring on claw health in lactating dairy cows housed in free-stall barns. J Dairy Sci 2006;89:4251–8.

10. Van Amstel SR, Shearer JK. Manual for the treatment and control of lameness in cattle. Ames (IA): Blackwell Publishing Professional; 2006. p. 59–125.

11. Greenough PR. Bovine laminitis and lameness, a hands-on approach. Elsevier Limited; 2007. p. 221–40.

12. Greenough PR, Weaver AD, Broom DM, et al. Basic concepts of bovine lameness. In: Greenough PR, Weaver AD, editors. Lameness in cattle. 3rd edition. RB Saunders; 1997.

13. Sprecher DJ, Hostetler DE, Kaneene JB. A lameness scoring system that uses posture and gait to predict dairy cattle reproductive performance. Theriogenology 1997;47:1178–87.

14. Desrochers A, Anderson DE, St-Jean G. Surgical treatment of lameness. Vet Clin North Am Food Anim Pract 2001;17(1):143–7.

15. Desrochers A. Upper leg lameness conditions. In: Proceedings of the AABP preconvention lameness seminar. September 19, 2007.

16. Shearer JK, Van Amstel SR. Pathophysiology and differentiation of toe lesions in dairy cattle. Proceedings of the Am College of Vet Int Med, June 9–10. Anaheim (CA). 2010. p. 253–5.

17. Van Amstel SR, Shearer JK, Palin FL. Moisture content, thickness, and lesions of sole horn associated with thin soles in dairy cattle. J Dairy Sci 2004;87: 757–63.

18. Shearer JK, van Amstel SR, Benzaquen M, et al. Effect of season on claw disorders (including thin soles) in a large dairy in the southeastern region of the United States. 14th Symposium on Lameness in Ruminants. Colonia del Sacramento (Uruguay): 2006. p. 110–1.

19. Van Amstel SR, Shearer JK, Palin FL, et al. The effect of parity, days in milk, season and walking surface on thin soles in dairy cattle. 14th International Symposium on Lameness in Ruminants. Colonia (Uruguay). 2006. p. 142–3.

20. Van Amstel SR, Shearer JK. Clinical Report – Characterization of toe ulcers associated with thin soles in dairy cows. Bovine Practitioner 2008;42(2):189–96.

21. Van Amstel S, Shearer JK. Approach to improve claw trimming in the southeastern United States. In: Lischer CJ, editor. Proceedings of the 10th Symposium on Lameness in Ruminants. Lucerne (Switzerland), September 7–10. 1998. p. 17.

22. Sanders AH, Shearer JK, DeVries A, et al. Seasonal incidence of lameness and risk factors associated with thin soles, white line disease, ulcers, and sole punctures in dairy cattle. J Dairy Sci 2009;92(7):3165–74.

23. Shearer J, Anderson D, Ayars W, Members of the Bovine Lameness Committee. A record-keeping system for the capture of lameness and foot care information in cattle. Bovine Practitioner 2004;38(1):83–92.

24. Cramer G, Lissemore KD, Guard CL, et al. Herd- and cow-level prevalence of foot lesions in Ontario dairy cattle. J Dairy Sci 2008;91:3888–95.

25. Kofler J, Hang A, Pesenhofer R, et al. Evaluation of claw health in heifers in seven dairy farms using a digital claw trimming protocol and claw data analysis system. Berl Munch Tierarztl Wochenschr 2011;124:272–81.

26. Van Amstel SR, Shearer JK. Review of Pododermatitis circumscripta (ulceration of the sole) in dairy cows. J Vet Intern Med 2006;20(4):805–11.

27. Vermunt JJ, Leach DH. A scanning electron microscopic study of the vascular system of the bovine hind limb claw. N Z Vet J 1992;40(4):146–54.

28. Danscher AM, Enemark JM, Telezhenko E, et al. Oligofructose overload induces lameness in cattle. J Dairy Sci 2009;92:607–16.

29. Rebhun WC, Payne RM, King JM, et al. Interdigital papillomatosis in dairy cattle. J Am Vet Med Assoc 1980;177:437–40.

30. Read DH, Walker RL. Papillomatous digital dermatitis (footwarts) in California dairy cattle: clinical and gross pathologic findings. J Vet Diagn Invest 1998;10:67–76.

31. Trott DJ, Moeller MR, Zuerner RL, et al. Characterization of Treponema phagedenis-like spirochetes isolated from papillomatous digital dermatitis lesions in dairy cattle. J Clin Microbiol 2003;41:2522–9.

32. Gomez A, Cook NB, Bernardoni ND, et al. An experimental infection model to induce digital dermatitis infection in cattle. J Dairy Sci 2012;95:1821–30.

33. Berry SL, Read DH, Walker RL, et al. Clinical, histologic, and bacteriologic findings in dairy cows with digital dermatitis (footwarts) one month after topical treatment with lincomycin hydrochloride or oxytetracycline hydrochloride. J Am Vet Med Assoc 2010;237:555–60.

34. Guard C. Lameness above the digit. In: Proceedings of the 2000 Hoof Health Conference. Duluth (MN). July 19–22. p. 22–3.

35. Sisson SB, Grossman JD. Bovine nervous system. In: The anatomy of domestic animals, 4th edition. WB Saunders, Philadelphia.

36. Smith–Maxie L. Pheripheral nerve diseases. In: Greenough PR, editor. Lameness in cattle. Philadelphia: WB Saunders; 1997. p. 203–18.

37. Kofler J. Ultrasonography as a diagnostic aid in bovine musculoskeletal disorders. In: Smith RA, Buczinski S, editors. 2009;(29)3:687–752.

38. Anderson DE, Desrochers A, StJean G. Management of tendon disorders in cattle. Vet Clin N Am Food Anim Pract 2008;3:551–66.

39. Nelson DR, Kneller SK. Treatment of proximal hind-limb lameness in cattle. Vet Clin N Am Food Anim Pract WB Saunders, Philadelphia. 1985; (1)1: 153–173.

40. Weaver AD. Spastic paresis and Downer cow. In: Greenough PR, editor. Lameness in cattle. Philadelphia: WB Saunders; 1997. p. p203–18.

41. Anderson DE. Lameness examination in cattle. In: Proceedings of the AABP preconvention lameness seminar. St Louis (MO). September 21, 2011.

Ruminant Toxicology Diagnostics

Steve Ensley, DVM, PhD*, Wilson Rumbeiha, DVM, PhD

KEYWORDS

- Toxicology • Analytical capability • Ruminants • Diagnostics

KEY POINTS

- The most common sources of ruminant poisoning are feed and water.
- Diagnoses of intoxications are based on history, clinical signs, lesions, laboratory examinations, and analytical chemistry.
- A complete history is necessary for developing the scheme of laboratory investigation and may be valuable in case of litigation.
- Many cases of ruminant toxicosis involve large numbers of animals affected acutely.

The most common sources of ruminant poisoning are feed and water. When confronted with a case of poisoning in ruminants, detailed examination of the environment and asking good questions of the animal caretakers should provide clues. Diagnoses of intoxications are based on history, clinical signs, lesions, laboratory examinations, and analytical chemistry. Circumstantial evidence is valuable and should be noted but does not replace a thorough clinical and postmortem examination. Histories from producers need to be viewed with scrutiny. A history of sudden death may actually mean that the producer just now found their animals dead.

Pertinent data and samples should be submitted to the diagnostic laboratory. A complete history is necessary for developing the scheme of laboratory investigation and may be valuable in case of litigation. Information should be detailed. For example, a notation of central nervous system (CNS) signs is not adequate; details of clinical signs should be described. Pertinent information that should be examined in the course of an investigation include: (1) the number of animals exposed or sick or dead, age, weight, and a chronology of morbidity and mortality; (2) clinical signs and course of the disease; (3) any prior disease conditions; (4) lesions observed at necropsy, with careful examination of ingesta; (5) response to treatment (medication should be listed to avoid analytic confusion); (6) related events, such as, feed change, water source, other medications, feed additives, pesticide applications; (7) description of facilities (a drawing or digital photograph may be helpful), access to refuse,

The authors have nothing to disclose.
Veterinary Diagnostic Laboratory, College of Veterinary Medicine, Iowa State University, Ames, IA 50011, USA
* Corresponding author.
E-mail address: sensley@iastate.edu

machinery, and so forth; and (8) recent past locations and when moved. The diagnostic laboratory should be contacted if there are questions regarding the appropriate sample, amount, or container.

Many cases of ruminant toxicosis involve large numbers of animals affected acutely. In some cases, large numbers of adult gazing animals are found dead on pasture. When death loss occurs in adult ruminants on pasture, the history is critical. Many times the animals are found dead or dying without any clinical signs observed before death. Having knowledge of what happens in a production setting at that particular time of the year is key information.

CASE 1: ADULT BEEF COWS DYING IN THE SPRING

Once infectious disease is ruled out in any case, toxicology issues moves up the rule-out list. Most veterinarians are more comfortable working through infectious disease scenarios because that is encountered most commonly. When adult beef cows are dying in the spring during calving, mineral-related issues such as calcium, magnesium, phosphorus, and potassium must be ruled out. Lactating animals are most prone to mineral deficiency and may die suddenly. Depending on the diet, these minerals may not be available at optimum concentrations in rations. Obtaining serum from affected animals before treatment is one method of determining mineral status. If it is not possible to obtain serum antemortem, ocular fluid or urine from dead animals may be used. Ocular magnesium concentration approximates serum values; ocular calcium is approximately 80% of serum values, whereas phosphorus and potassium values can be variable.[1-16] Fertilization of forages with elevated concentrations of potassium interferes with absorption of magnesium from the diet. Knowing forage concentration is helpful. High potassium forages can develop when pastures are fertilized with nitrogen, phosphorus, and potassium to obtain optimum yields of forage. Such heavily fertilized pastures are also high risk for nitrate poisoning.

If ocular concentrations of macrominerals are within normal limits, additional analysis may be performed. This includes determination of nitrate and/or nitrite and ammonia nitrogen concentration.

Criteria used to determine excess nitrate exposure in ruminants include

1. Signs of oxygen deprivation
2. Evidence of chocolate-colored blood or tissues
3. Elevated nitrate and/or nitrite concentrations in serum, blood, plasma, forages, or ocular fluid.

Although both nitrate and nitrite have a relatively short half-life in blood, nitrate has a longer half-life than nitrite; therefore, nitrate can consistently be used to determine excess exposure to high nitrate diets. Specimens need to be collected and refrigerated or frozen. Ocular fluid nitrate and/or nitrite concentrations correlate with serum values. Ocular fluid remains stable for 24 hours at room temperature and 1 week refrigerated. Serum and ocular fluid values helpful for diagnosis of toxicosis in animals are greater than 20 ppm nitrate and greater than 0.5 ppm nitrite.[17-23]

If pregnant ruminants are exposed to excess nitrate and/or nitrite concentration in the diet or water, abortions may follow. Fetuses are more sensitive to nitrate poisoning than dams.[17-23]

The following criteria can be used to diagnose a fetal abortion with excessive nitrate exposure:

1. Clinical signs of nitrate toxicosis in the dam
2. Abortion within 1 to 2 weeks after onset of diagnosed toxicosis in the surviving dams

3. Concurrent fetal ocular fluid nitrate and nitrite content greater than 40 ppm nitrate and greater than 0.5 ppm nitrite/mL[17-23]: ocular fluid is the most ideal specimen in dead animals, but it can also be contaminated by bacteria; bacterial contamination of ocular fluid produces nitric oxide, which converts to nitrate and/or nitrite (chemical analysis cannot differentiate between exogenous and endogenous nitrate and nitrite)
4. Detection of elevated nitrate in feed and/or forage or water that supports a diagnosis of an acute nitrate toxicosis in the dam: forage nitrate greater than 10,000 ppm nitrate on a dry matter basis and water greater than 450 ppm nitrate.[17-23]

If ruminants are exposed to excess nonprotein nitrogen (NPN) sources toxicosis may result. Also, animals lose adaptability to NPN rather quickly. So toxicosis may arise from exposure to high normal NPN in feeds if supplements ran out for as few as 2 to 3 days. Urea is the most common NPN with biuret, urea phosphate, ammonia polyphosphate, diammonium phosphate, monoammonium phosphate, and ammonium acetate also being used as an NPN source. NPN sources are hydrolyzed to ammonia (NH_3) in the rumen. When the rumen pH is lower than seven, ammonia is converted into ammonium (NH_4+) through the addition of a proton. Ammonium does not move easily across the rumen wall and is not easily absorbed into the blood stream. As ammonium accumulates in the rumen, the rumen pH increases. As the rumen pH increases, the conversion to ammonium slows down and the reaction shifts back to the production of ammonia. The ammonia is readily absorbed across the rumen wall into the circulation where it is converted into urea by the liver.[24] When the liver becomes overwhelmed by excess ammonia in the bloodstream, an ammonia toxicosis occurs. Analysis for ammonia nitrogen (NH_3N) can be performed on rumen fluid, CNS fluid, ocular fluid, serum, or whole blood. The feed can also be analyzed for NPN. Finding elevations in any of the animal fluids is needed for diagnosis of ammonia toxicosis. Postmortem changes can interfere with diagnosis. The rumen pH typically decreases after death. In addition, autolysis produces ammonia, complicating diagnosis. Depending on environmental conditions, obtaining an adequate sample to analyze for ammonia nitrogen may be difficult. It is important to analyze samples immediately, preferably within 6 hours, to avoid inaccurate test results caused by deterioration of samples (**Table 1**).

In cases involving acute death, determination of exposure of animals to organophosphates or carbamates is also important in the differential diagnosis. Determining exposure to organophosphates or carbamates is done by measuring acetylcholinesterase (AChE) activity. There are several different methods to determine AChE, so a veterinarian must check with the laboratory conducting the testing to determine the method and the concentration guidelines they use. In the authors' laboratory, we prefer to measure AChE activity in the caudate nucleus of the brain. The primary purpose of measuring this area is to provide a consistent area of the brain that is sampled. There is data to indicate that the caudate nucleus may contain the highest

Table 1		
	Normal Concentration	**Elevated Concentration**
Rumen fluid	<80 mg/dL	>80 mg/dL
Vitreous	<0.5 mg/dL	>1 mg/dL
CNS, serum, blood	<0.5 mg/dL	>1 mg/dL

Data from Plumlee K. Clinical veterinary toxicology. St Louis (MO): Mosby; 2004.

concentration of AChE in the brain for the longest period postmortem.[25–27] One caveat with AChE assays is that they are affected by sample integrity. Autolyzed tissues yield a false negative test result. For this reason, we prefer actual detection and identification of the pesticide in rumen contents, liver, fat, and feeds. This can be done using gas chromatography mass spectrometry analysis on fresh or frozen samples. **Table 2** Detection of organophosphate or carbamate compounds with consistent clinical signs is a more definitive diagnosis that relying on AChE activity alone.

CASE 2: DETERMINATION OF MINERAL STATUS IN RUMINANTS

Measuring the mineral status of ruminants is often of interest to veterinarians and producers. Veterinary toxicology laboratories have become involved in determining trace mineral concentrations in ruminants because many cases involve excesses or deficiencies. Determining mineral status has been used to assist in evaluating the health of ruminants. A recent improvement in instrumentation in the chemistry laboratory has allowed multiple trace minerals to be evaluated at once, thus reducing the cost. This method involves the use of inductively coupled plasma to determine mineral status.

Trace minerals are defined as any chemical element required by living organisms in minute amounts. This definition is not exact. Exact mineral needs vary among species. Macrominerals are defined as minerals required in the diet in relatively large amounts. They include calcium, phosphorus, potassium, sodium, chloride, magnesium, and zinc. In ruminants, trace minerals of interest that have been studied include cobalt, copper, iodine, iron, manganese, molybdenum, selenium, and zinc. Trace minerals measured but difficult to interpret include aluminum, antimony, barium, beryllium,

Table 2
Toxicant and/or analyte and handling

Toxicant and/or Analyte	Sample of Choice	Handling and Submitting Samples
Acetylcholinesterase	Whole blood, fresh brain	Refrigerate blood, refrigerate or freeze brain
Nitrate and/or nitrite	Ocular fluid or serum	Remove fluid from the eye and refrigerate or freeze, refrigerate or freeze serum
Nitrate and/or nitrite	Feed or water	Collect a representative sample and refrigerate
Cyanide	Feed	Collect a representative sample and refrigerate
NPN	Ocular fluid, serum, rumen content	Remove fluid from the eye and freeze, freeze serum and rumen content rapidly
Ionophores	Retained feed sample from the feed at the time of exposure	Dry, room temperature
Trace mineral	Serum or liver	Refrigerate or freeze serum or liver
Gas Chromatography Mass Spectroscopy	Blood, serum, urine, rumen content, tissue	Refrigerate or freeze except whole blood, which is not frozen

boron, lithium, nickel, platinum, rhenium, silicon, silver, strontium, sulfur, thallium, tin, titanium, and vanadium.[28] Just because a mineral can be measured does not mean it can be interpreted. Minerals required for animal diets depend on the animal and type of production. The needs are different depending on whether the animal is pregnant or lactating, growing or finishing, a steer or a heifer, and so forth. Minerals required also depend on the geographic area. Serum samples in general represent what the animal's diet has been for the previous week. Liver samples in general represent what the animal's diet has been for the last month. When serum mineral samples are evaluated, an increased or decreased value is meaningful. Depending on the mineral, a normal value for a serum mineral may not necessarily mean that the animal has adequate mineral status. For example, in the case of copper, the liver may be depleted, but the animal maintains a normal serum concentration as long as it is able. Trace mineral concentrations are easier to interpret from liver samples because it is the storage organ for trace minerals.

A class of elements that is a major concern is the heavy metals. There is no exact scientific definition of what a heavy metal is and there is some confusion over heavy versus toxic metals. The elements typically included in a heavy (toxic) metal panel include antimony, arsenic, beryllium, cadmium, chromium, lead, mercury, nickel, selenium, thallium, and vanadium.[24] The authors' laboratory offers a toxic heavy metal panel that includes all the above elements. Different laboratories offer different configurations of panels. Heavy metals have little nutritional value if any, but cause intoxication at relatively low concentrations.

CASE 3: UNKNOWN CAUSE OF DEATH IN MULTIPLE ANIMALS

Veterinary diagnosticians may be presented with cases with very little history other than sudden death of several previously healthy animals. An accurate history is essential; potential infectious causes of the adverse effect should be ruled out before the focus turns to toxicology. For diagnostic testing it is prudent to start out with the most inexpensive and most pertinent analysis available. These include previously discussed tests such as nitrate, determination of cholinesterase activity, and ammonia nitrogen concentration. If these analyses are within normal limits, the next step is to determine the presence of any heavy metals in the liver. If analyses are negative up to this point, then a gas chromatograph–mass spectroscopy (GC-MS) screen can be initiated. Samples can be analyzed for pesticides (organochlorines, organophosphates, or carbamates), aliphatic hydrocarbons, industrial pollutants, disinfectants, oxidants other miscellaneous pesticides, polycyclic aromatics, alkyl benzenes, some anticoagulant compounds, some natural products, vitamins, some plant and fungal toxins, and some drugs. The GC-MS contains a library of chemical profiles that can be matched to an unknown organic compound for identification. Not all cases involving toxicants are solved satisfactorily but, using the tools available, many can be.

CASE 4: IONOPHORE TOXICOSIS

Ionophores are a common feed additive for ruminants and, when fed according to the label instructions, are very safe. When there is a significant dosing error with ionophores, toxicosis may develop. A one-time dosing error can cause adverse effects that may continue for weeks to months. Typically, when there is ionophore intoxication, the first clinical sign is anorexia or feed refusal. Anorexia may develop within hours and within 12–24 hours there is diarrhea. Death loss in ruminants normally does not occur immediately after the dosing error. The first death loss is usually 2 to 3 days after the overdose, complicating diagnosis. At the time of the first death loss and before the realization that there was an overdose, adulterated feed is usually continually fed. Frequently, the offending feed is finished feeding before clinical signs manifest. Feed analysis can be helpful for a diagnosis even though ionophores have a relatively short half-life. When an animal goes off feed and dies 3 days after consuming a toxic dose, consumption of the feed with elevated ionophores ceases within twenty four hours of the over dose. There is little likelihood that any of the ionophore will be detected in the rumen content at the time of death. The time line of exposure and death is helpful in diagnosis. After exposure, death loss typically starts in 2 to 3 days with a peak in death loss at 7 to 10 days after the over dose. Death loss can continue for weeks to months after the over dose; therefore, all death loss in affected cattle must be investigated to determine cause of death. The cause of extended death loss after an acute over dose of an ionophore is cardiac necrosis and resulting fibrosis and the resultant heart failure. Determining ante-mortem after an acute exposure which animals in a pen have enough cardiac damage to die is difficult. Many times animals appear healthy and are eating but are found suddenly dead hours later. Pen riders and animal caretakers become frustrated because of the acute death of affected animals. Do not assume that all death loss in a pen is due to iono-phore toxicosis after an acute overdose. Animals may die from other causes. It is advis-able to collect tissues from animals that die in a pen that has been overdosed from an ionophore and retain these in formalin to examine microscopically if needed to deter-mine the full extent of death loss due to ionophores. To diagnose ionophore toxicosis, it is useful to examine cardiac and skeletal muscle microscopically. The pathologic char-acteristics may be in either or in both of these muscles, depending on the species. The liver concentration of vitamin E and selenium should be determined because a deficiency of vitamin E and selenium are primary rule-outs. An overdose with gossypol can also cause cardiomyopathy. Animals in a confined feeding operation do not usually have access to any poisonous plants such as white snake root, which can also cause myopathy.

To summarize ionophore toxicosis: examining the appropriate cardiac and skeletal muscle for typical pathologic signs of ionophore toxicosis is more valuable than analyzing rumen contents. A feed analysis may be helpful but, more often, the offend-ing feed is finished by the time clinical signs show. Saving retained batches of feeds for possible analysis in the future may be helpful in many cases of toxicosis.

CASE 5: COPPER TOXICOSIS

Determining copper toxicosis in ruminants, especially sheep, is straightforward. The liver is the storage organ for copper. As copper accumulates in the liver it reaches a crit-ical concentration when the hepatocytes are no longer able to store the copper intra-cellularly. When this critical concentration is reached, under stressful triggering events the copper is suddenly released into the blood stream causing acute intravas-cular hemolysis. Measuring copper and kidney concentration in the liver usually provides the information needed to determine if the cause of death is copper toxicosis. Unless there is evidence of hemolysis, high liver copper concentrations alone are not sufficient to confirm a diagnosis of copper poisoning. Analysis of the kidney for elevated copper concentrations is helpful confirming a diagnosis of copper poisoning. Exam-ining the liver and kidney microscopically assists in diagnosis if the appropriate patho-logic lesions are observed. One of the remaining questions is: which other animals in this group have elevated liver copper and are at risk of death? Unfortunately, measuring the concentration of serum copper in the remaining animals does not reveal the liver concentration of copper accurately all the time. Frequently, the serum copper is within a normal range even when the liver is extremely elevated with copper or even slightly depleted. Performing a liver biopsy to determine liver copper concentration may stress an animal with elevated liver copper and cause death. Once copper toxicosis is diagnosed in an animal in a group, it is helpful to treat the remainder of the animals with elevated molybdenum in the feed for 1 month to help reduce copper absorption and deplete the copper from the liver.[24]

REFERENCES

1. Abbitt B. A case of nitrate-induced abortion in cattle. Southwestern Veterinarian 1982;35(1):12.
2. Allsop TF, Pauli JV. Magnesium concentrations in the ventricular and lumbar cerebrospinal fluid of hypomagnesaemic cows. Res Vet Sci 1985;38:61–4.
3. Drolet R, D'Allaire S, Chagnon M. The evaluation of postmortem ocular fluid analysis as a diagnostic aid in sows. J Vet Diagn Invest 1990;2:9–13.
4. Edwards G, Foster A, Livesey C. Use of ocular fluids to aid postmortem diagnosis in cattle and sheep. Practice 2009;31:22–5.
5. Haggard DL, Whitehair CK, Langham RF. Tetany associated with magnesium deficiency in suckling beef calves. J Am Vet Med Assoc 1978;172:495–7.
6. Hall RF, Reynolds RA. Concentrations of magnesium and calcium in plasma of Hereford cows during and after hypomagnesemic tetany. Am J Vet Res 1972;33:1711–3.
7. Hanna P, Bellamy J, Donald A. Postmortem eyefluid analysis in dogs, cats and cattle as an estimate of antemortem serum chemistry profiles. Can J Vet Res 1990;54:487–94.
8. Hazel S, Thrall M, Severin G, et al. Laboratory evaluation of aqueous humor in the healthy dog, cat, horse and cow. Am J Vet Res 1985;46:657–9.
9. McCoy MA. Hypomagnesaemia and new data on vitreous humour magnesium concentration as a post-mortem marker in ruminants. Magnes Res 2004;17:137–45.
10. McCoy MA, Bingham V, Hudson AJ, et al. Postmortem biochemical markers of experimentally induced hypomagnesaemic tetany in sheep. Vet Rec 2001;148:233–7.
11. McCoy MA, Hudson AJ, Hutchinson T, et al. Postsampling stability of eye fluid magnesium concentrations in cattle. Vet Rec 2001;148:312–3.
12. McCoy MA, Hutchinson T, Davison G, et al. Postmortem biochemical markers of experimentally induced hypomagnesaemic tetany in cattle. Vet Rec 2001;148:268–73.
13. McLaughlin B, McLaughlin P. Equine vitreous humor chemical concentrations: correlation with serum concentrations, and postmortem changes with time and temperature. Can J Vet Res 1988;52:476–80.
14. McLaughlin P, McLaughlin B. Chemical analysis of bovine and porcine vitreous humors: correlation of normal values with serum chemical values and changes with time and temperature. Am J Vet Res 1987;48:467–73.
15. Mulei CM, Daniel RC. The effect of induced hypomagnesaemia and hypermagnesaemia on the erythrocyte magnesium concentration in cattle. Vet Res Commun 1988;12:289–93.
16. Odette O. Grass tetany in a herd of beef cows. Can Vet J 2005;46:732–4.
17. Johnson J, Grotelueschen D, Knott T. Evaluation of bovine perinatal nitrate accumulation in western Nebraska. Vet Hum Toxicol 1994;36:467–71.
18. Johnson J, Schneider N, Kelling C, et al. Nitrate exposure in perinatal beef calves. The 26th Annual Meeting of the American Association of Veterinary Laboratory Diagnosticians. 1983; p. 167–80.

19. Boermans H. Diagnosis of nitrate toxicosis in cattle using biological fluids and a rapid ion chromatographic method. Am J Vet Res 1990;51:491.
20. Carlson M. The distribution of nitrate and nitrite in the pregnant cow, and endogenous production of nitrate and nitrite by stimulated macrophages. Omaha (NE): University of Nebraska Medical Center; 1996.
21. Hibbs C, Stencel E, Hill R. Nitrate toxicosis in cattle. Vet Hum Toxicol 1978;20:1–2.
22. Hudson D, Rawls J. Nitrate toxicity in a commercial beef herd. Nebraska Cattleman 1992;48(7):58.
23. Wood P. The molecular pathology of chronic nitrate intoxication in domestic animals: a hypothesis. Vet Hum Toxicol 1980;22:26–7.
24. Plumlee K. Clinical veterinary toxicology. St Louis (MO): Mosby; 2004.
25. Carson TL, Furr AA. Interpretation of blood and brain cholinesterase values in organophosphate/carbamate insecticide poisoning in cattle and sheep. 19th Annual Proceedings American Association of Veterinary Laboratory Diagnosticians. 1976; p. 305–10.
26. Morgan S, Martin T. Determination of cholinesterase levels in cerebrum and caudate nucleus from 100 normal cattle. Vet Hum Toxicol 1986;28(5):417.
27. Mount M, Oehme F. Brain cholinesterase activity in healthy cattle, swine and sheep exposed to cholinesterase inhibiting insecticides. Am J Vet Res 1981; 42:1345–50.
28. Kincaid RL. Assessment of trace mineral status of ruminants: a review. Proceedings of the American Society of Animal Science. 1999; p. 1–10.

Molecular Diagnostics Applied to Mastitis Problems on Dairy Farms

Abhijit Gurjar, DVM, PhD[a],*, Gloria Gioia, PhD[a,b],
Ynte Schukken, DVM, PhD[a], Frank Welcome, DVM, MBA[a],
Ruth Zadoks, DVM, PhD[a,c], Paolo Moroni, DVM, PhD[a,d]

KEYWORDS

- Mastitis • Molecular diagnostics • *Staphylococcus aureus* • *Mycoplasma bovis*
- *Streptococcus uberis* • *Enterobacter*

KEY POINTS

- In the last decade, molecular diagnostics have been added to the toolkit of the mastitis researcher community.
- The choice of a molecular typing method depends on the needs, skill level, and resources of the laboratory.
- Many bacterial species have a large genetic variation and within a species many strains exist that have very different infection characteristics in the bovine mammary gland and epidemiologic characteristics within a herd.
- Accurate and cost-effective methods of identifying mastitis pathogens are important for the diagnosis, surveillance, and control of this economically important disease among dairy cows.

INTRODUCTION

Mastitis in dairy cows is among the most important diseases of dairy cattle worldwide. Mastitis is most often the response of the host to an intramammary infection (IMI) and is caused by a large number of bacterial species.[1] Accurate and cost-effective methods of identifying mastitis pathogens are important for the diagnosis, surveillance, and control of this economically important disease among dairy cows. Rapid identification methods, in particular nucleic acid–based tests, have the potential to be extremely specific and can also discriminate among closely related organisms.[2]

The authors have nothing to disclose.

[a] Quality Milk Production Services, College of Veterinary Medicine, Cornell University, 240 Farrier Road, Ithaca, NY 14853, USA; [b] Department of Veterinary Science and Public Health, Università degli Studi di Milano, via Celoria 10, Milan 20133, Italy; [c] Moredun Research Institute, Pentlands Science Park, Bush Loan, Penicuik, Midlothian EH26 0PZ, Scotland; [d] Department of Health, Animal Science and Food Safety, Università degli Studi di Milano, Milan 20133, Italy
* Corresponding author.
E-mail address: aag88@cornell.edu

Vet Clin Food Anim 28 (2012) 565–576
http://dx.doi.org/10.1016/j.cvfa.2012.07.011
0749-0720/12/$ – see front matter Published by Elsevier Inc.

vetfood.theclinics.com

The development of diagnostic and monitoring tools is experiencing an unprecedented growth phase. In the last decade, molecular diagnostics have been added to the toolkit of the mastitis researcher community.[3] These new tools have resulted in a better understanding of epidemiology and pathobiology of IMI. The goal of molecular epidemiology, however, is not merely to classify organisms into taxonomic or phylogenetic groups but also to "identify the microparasites responsible for the infectious diseases and determine their physical sources, their biologic relationships, and their route of transmission and those of genes responsible for their virulence, vaccine-relevant antigens and drug resistance."[4]

STRAIN TYPING METHODS

These molecular methods include comparative typing methods, library typing methods, virulence gene arrays, and whole-genome sequencing.[5] This article describes the relationship among the epidemiology of some major bacterial infections of the mammary gland using molecular diagnostic techniques. The ideal diagnostic technique should be cost-effective and easy to perform. Its results should preserve a balance between increased discriminating power and applicability. Rapid identification methods, in particular nucleic acid–based tests, have the potential to be extremely specific and can also discriminate among closely related organisms.[2]

The process of subtyping is important epidemiologically for recognizing outbreaks of infection, detecting the transmission of nosocomial pathogens, determining the source of the infection, and recognizing particularly virulent strains of organisms.[6] Any subtyping method must have high differentiation power. It must be able to clearly differentiate unrelated strains, such as those that are geographically distinct from the source organism, and at the same time to demonstrate the genetic relationship of all organisms isolated from individuals infected through the same source.[7]

Many of the currently used molecular techniques for typing rely on electrophoretic separation of DNA fragments of different molecular lengths. The electrophoretic result is represented by a pattern of bands on a gel. Because these patterns may be extremely complex, the ease with which the patterns are interpreted and related is an important factor in evaluating the use of a particular typing method. Along with considerations related to a particular method's simplicity of interpretation, its convenience of use is also important. The technical difficulty, cost, and time to obtain a result must also be evaluated in assessing the use of a particular typing method. The choice of a molecular typing method depends on the needs, skill level, and resources of the laboratory.

Currently, sequencing of RNA or DNA is routinely used for molecular typing. Such methodologies allow for the sequence data to be available for whole genomes or selected areas, such as specific genes or repetitive elements. A major advantage of sequence data is that it is unambiguous, and can easily be stored and exchanged.[2]

In contrast, in the comparative typing methods, such as random amplification polymorphic DNA (RAPD) and pulse field gel electrophoresis, band sizes need to be expressed relative to each other. Many sequence-based typing methods and hybrids of banding pattern and sequences-based methods exist, and it is beyond the scope of this article to discuss all of them.

PRIMARY DIAGNOSIS OF PATHOGENS

A wide range of DNA-based diagnostic assays have been developed and applied to the diagnosis of bovine IMI, and for the improved detection of pathogens in milk and animal feed.[8] These techniques have changed the molecular diagnostic scene and must be considered as one of the more important developments during the last few years. Compared with the classical bacteriologic diagnosis the molecular technologies offer several important, well-known advantages, such as faster and higher throughput assays, lower costs per detected agent, if the equipment can be used for a large number of samples, and ability to differentiate between clonal outbreak and multiple strains. Particularly, real-time (RT) polymerase chain reaction (PCR) assays offer several important, well-known advantages:

1. Faster and higher throughput assays
2. Post-PCR handling of the amplicons/products is not required and hands-on time is greatly reduced compared with traditional detection using agarose gels followed by ethidium bromide staining
3. Probes can be labeled with several different fluorophores that function as individual reporter dyes for different primer sets; thus, it is suitable for the development of multiplex PCR systems
4. Lower costs per detected agent, if the equipment can be used for a large number of samples

Diagnostics of selected mastitis pathogens is likely an attractive application of the RT-PCR technology.

OBJECTIVES OF THIS ARTICLE

This article highlights the application in several real farm case studies of routinely used molecular techniques for primary diagnosis and epidemiologic investigation of IMI caused by major mastitis pathogens, such as *Staphylococcus aureus*, *Mycoplasma bovis*, *Streptococcus uberis*, and *Enterobacter* spp.

Staphylococcus aureus

Staphylococcus aureus is an important organism isolated in subclinical and chronic mastitis in bovines.[9] Bovine mastitis caused by *S aureus* inflicts enormous economic loss on dairy farms and is characterized by persistent and contagious in nature. Some strains of *S aureus* demonstrate antibiotic resistance and may persist for longer periods without overt symptoms. The diagnosis, surveillance, and control of this economically important mastitis pathogen are based on accurate, rapid, and cost-effective methods of identifying the pathogen. To formulate effective strategies for reducing the spread of *S aureus* infection it is very important to understand the distribution of the pathogen in dairy herds.[10] Various phenotyping techniques, such as biotyping, bacteriophage typing, and antibiotic sensitivity testing, have been routinely used in different epidemiologic studies of *S aureus* isolated from human and animal populations.[7,11] The use of phenotyping methods could be expensive, time consuming, and subject to considerable variation.[12] One of the genotyping method used extensively to fingerprint strains of various microorganisms is RAPD. The technique uses single, short, random sequence oligonucleotide primers resulting in discrete and characteristic patterns of DNA fragments.[12] The profiles obtained after electrophoretic separation of the amplified DNA fragments can be used to study the genetic diversity and structure of the natural population of a number of human and animal pathogens. The RAPD technique is rapid and discriminatory.[13]

Epidemiologic studies involving genotyping of strains from host and the environment are necessary to establish effective preventive measures in the spread of *S aureus* involved in IMI. The case study presented in this article describes the use of RAPD technique to determine the genetic relatedness of *S aureus* associated with bovine IMIs in a dairy herd. The *S aureus* isolates came from an approximately 2000-cow dairy farm that had a low bulk milk somatic cell count at approximately 150,000 cells/mL. Data analysis of the farm indicated that based on individual cow somatic cell count data the average infection duration was approximately 2 months (cure risk was approximately 50%; average duration, in test day intervals, is estimated as the inverse of the cure risk); a low risk of new infections at approximately 5%; and clinical mastitis that was most prominent immediately after calving. This analysis of the herd data pointed more toward a noncontagious infection pattern than toward a classical contagious transmission pattern. The infection profile from clinical mastitis samples showed a large variety in the number of bacterial species causing IMIs without a predominance of a single bacterial species. Among the bacterial species was a relatively large number of *S aureus* isolates, and given the classical connection between *S aureus* and contagious transmission, the owner of the farm was concerned about a potential mastitis outbreak caused by *S aureus* and was determined to change milking procedures and overhaul his milking equipment. A farm risk assessment was performed and no major deficiency in milking procedures or functioning of the milking equipment was observed. Cow cleanliness was an issue and the use of sprinkler systems in the summer resulted in many teats dripping with water before entering the milking parlor. Therefore, risk assessment pointed more toward a high environmental infection risk rather than contagious transmission risk.

A total of 54 *S aureus* isolates were analyzed using RAPD. Briefly, amplification reactions were performed in 20-μL volumes containing 10 μL of GoTaq Green Mastermix (Promega WI, USA); 7 μL of water; 1 μL of 10-bp oligonucleotide primers AAG3 (5′-GGGACGGCCA-3′); and 2 μL of template DNA. The amplification consisted of initial denaturation at 95°C for 5 minutes, followed by 45 cycles of 30 seconds at 94°C, 1 minute at 35°C, and 2 minutes at 72°C. A final extension step of 72°C for 5 minutes was included in all amplifications.

Out of the total 54 *S aureus* isolates 16 (30%) came from composite string milk samples, and the remaining 38 (70%) came from individual quarter milk samples. Amplification of the *S aureus* isolates by RAPD technique resulted in a polymorphic pattern composed of 8 to 12 clear bands in the range 200 to more than 2000 bp (**Fig. 1**). In the current case report, we found that identification of genetic diversity in *S aureus* strains from the farm (see **Fig. 1**) was primarily related to the problem of many different *S aureus* strains on the farm. In our study we identified eight common RAPD strain types and 46 distinct RAPD profiles. This fact suggests that for these eight clonal isolates, there may be a common source of *S aureus* in this herd. The results for the remaining isolates indicate a nonclonal transmission pattern of *S aureus* on this dairy farm. Communication back to the dairy producer emphasized the noncontagious nature of the *S aureus* IMI in this herd. It was advised to segregate the known infected cows, apply treatment to young animals with a recent infection, eventually cull older and long-term infected animals, and continue the excellent milking practices that have prevented infection transmission of the *S aureus* strains in the herd. In conclusion, molecular typing of the identified *S aureus* isolates showed a nonclonal infection transmission pattern. With this additional information on top of the species determination (*S aureus*), much more precise and accurate advice could be provided to the farm manager.

RAPD was a useful technique for distinguishing strains within species of *S aureus*. This technique provides useful information for understanding molecular epidemiology of *S aureus* within dairy herds and more specifically for investigating the source of *S aureus* mastitis outbreaks, thereby contributing to better management of *S aureus* mastitis in dairy herds.

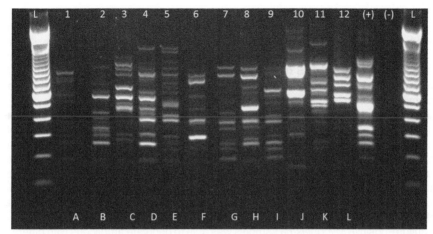

Fig. 1. RAPD gel showing a nonclonal outbreak of *Staphylococcus aureus* in 12 cows in a New York dairy farm. Mastitis isolates of *S aureus* from the farm are in lanes 1 to 12. Lanes coded with (+), (−), and L are positive and negative controls and DNA ladder, respectively.

Mycoplasma spp

Mycoplasma bovis, with increased cattle movement over recent years, is the most common disease implicated in pneumonia and mastitis.[14] Despite this, there is still poor appreciation of its impact on animal health and welfare, with underdiagnosis in many countries because of a lack of the specialized techniques required to detect the organism and incomplete understanding of the pathogenesis of infection. The standard laboratory diagnosis for mycoplasma mastitis is currently based on microbiologic procedures by bacterial isolation from bulk tank milk or samples from cows with clinical and subclinical mastitis. Over recent years enzyme-linked immunosorbent assay and PCR-based methods have gradually replaced culture as the method of choice for detecting *M bovis*, and the application of a novel RT-PCR method makes a valuable new contribution in this context.[15,16] Diagnosis for mycoplasma using cultures has intrinsic limitations in terms of sensitivity and test turnaround time and it is not expected that these drawbacks will be overcome by significant improvements in culture-based methods in the near future. The isolation and subsequent subculturing for mycoplasma identification is a time-consuming process that may take up to 15 days before a sample is considered negative or positive for mycoplasma.[17] In addition to a significant time delay in detection, the traditional culture-based methods often fail to isolate mycoplasmas because the viability of the organism declines rapidly during transport and storage.[18]

Early detection of mycoplasma infections is important in preventing disease and reducing the spread to other animals; in this regard it is essential to develop laboratory methods faster than the traditional bacteriologic approach. The routine mycoplasma diagnosis may also be based on serologic and biochemical assays, but it is well documented that these microorganisms share common surface components responsible for cross-reactivity.[19] In addition to this it has been observed that mycoplasma have the ability to vary their size, shape, and surface antigens further complicating identification by these techniques.[20] The molecular approaches represent a valid and promising option to overcome these limits. However, reliability and sensitivity of these methods are highly dependent on the extraction of adequate amounts of pure DNA using appropriate methods (Gioia, personal communication, 2012).

The molecular epidemiology of mastitis-associated *Mycoplasma* spp has been investigated by such approaches as Amplified Fragment Length Polymorphism (AFLP), pulse field gel electrophoresis, and restriction enzyme typing analysis.[3] The PCR assays for the detection of mycoplasma are mostly based on in vitro amplification of the highly conserved 16S rRNA gene. However, PCR tests developed on the 16S target without further sequences analysis fail to differentiate among different *Mycoplasma* species.[21]

The low degree of variation in the 16S rRNA gene sequences suggests a potential misdiagnosis using only 16S rRNA-based PCR assays. Subramaniam and colleagues[22] developed a PCR based on the DNA repair *uvrC* gene, which was shown to clearly differentiate between *M bovis* and other *Mycoplasma* species. The authors recently developed a single-step duplex PCR assay using a combination of two primer pairs, one universal for *Mycoplasma* genus designed on the 16S target and one specific for *M bovis*, targeting the *uvrC* gene, thus allowing the simultaneous and unequivocal detection and differentiation *M bovis* from other *Mycoplasma* spp. This assay performed on culture-positive *Mycoplasma* samples was able to generate amplicons with different size respectively for *Mycoplasma* spp and *M bovis*. The single-step multiplex PCR ensured high sensitivity and specificity with quick turnaround time for test results. The multiplex PCR assay represents an additional tool for epidemiologic studies and routine disease assessment in areas endemic for the multiple *Mycoplasma* species.

The represented case study is from a dairy herd of 600 Holstein milking cows with a mean daily milk production of 32 kg per cow per day. This dairy farm experienced a sudden increase in the incidence of respiratory problem in lactating heifers and after approximately 50 days the same animals showed signs of clinical mastitis. Forty-three cases of clinical mastitis were recorded over a 15-day period. During the outbreak, bacteriologic examination was performed on samples from clinically affected cows (including bulk tank milk and lungs). Identification of *Mycoplasma* infection and determination of the species *(M bovis)* was performed in one diagnostic procedure with the developed duplex PCR (**Fig. 2**). Early detection of the *M bovis* from the submitted samples assisted in quick diagnosis and management of *Mycoplasma* outbreak in this herd. Cows were segregated immediately and culled where possible. Appropriate

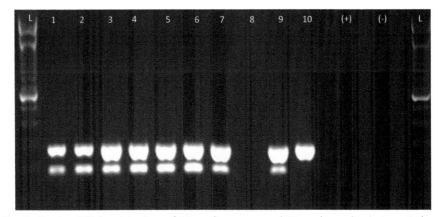

Fig. 2. Duplex PCR for detection of *Mycoplasma* spp and *Mycoplasma bovis*. Lane 1, lung sample positive for *M bovis*; lanes 2 to 7, milk samples positive for *M bovis*; lane 8, milk sample negative for *Mycoplasma*; lane 9, positive control to *M bovis* (ATCC 25523); lane 10, positive control to *Mycoplasma* spp (ATCC 29103); lanes coded with (+), (−), and L are positive and negative controls and DNA ladder, respectively.

management techniques were emphasized in the milk parlor and for the hospital pen. Because of quick diagnosis and immediate response, further expansion of the outbreak was halted.

This case study signifies the importance of application of a novel diagnostic tool, such as duplex PCR, for early detection and screening of *Mycoplasma* in a dairy herd thereby aiding in control and management of the outbreak.

Streptococcus uberis

Streptococcus uberis is a major mastitis-causing pathogen that is generally classified as an organism of environmental origin. *S uberis* has been associated with subclinical and clinical IMIs in lactating and nonlactating cows.[23] Typically, the authors classify *S uberis* as an environmental organism, meaning that infection occurs because of organisms in the environment of cows.[24] In the case of *S uberis*, one would therefore predict that most strains causing infections in a herd should be genotypically different because an enormous number of different genotypes of *S uberis* exist in the environment of the cow.[25] In some cases it has been observed that a single strain of *S uberis* caused mastitis in multiple cows.[26] This observation of a single strain in multiple IMIs would potentially indicate that transmission between animals occurs, and that the bacterium behaves more like a contagious organism.

RAPD fingerprinting has also been used for confirmation of *S uberis* after intramammary challenge with *S uberis* and identified new *S uberis* infections in challenged quarters. Subtyping of *S uberis* and *Streptococcus dysgalactiae* by RAPD fingerprinting demonstrated isolates from New Zealand were distinct from isolates from the United States.[12]

A 1700-cow dairy farm was concerned about an increase in *S uberis* clinical mastitis observed during a 3-month period. Clinical mastitis was observed in approximately 5% of cows on a monthly basis. The herd manager focused on improving stalls and cow hygiene given the classical environmental organisms observed in clinical cases (*S uberis* and coliforms). Subsequent data analysis and risk assessment on the farm pointed toward a high risk of transmission, particularly during milking. The authors observed that known infected cows were not segregated and postmilking teat disinfection was done with a spray system and showed very poor teat coverage with the disinfectant. Dynamic measurements of the milking equipment showed that there was a high fluctuation of vacuum under the teat-end. This high fluctuation of vacuum was caused by a low effective reserve relative to the size of the milking parlor.

Molecular methods were used for strain typing and to confirm the species identity of isolates that had been classified as *Streptococcus* spp based on phenotypic characteristics. Strain typing was performed using RAPD PCR. Briefly, crude DNA extracts from *S uberis* isolates were obtained by 10-minute boil preparation and used as templates for RAPD PCR with primer set OPE-04 (5k-GTGACATGCC-3k; Operon Technologies, Alameda, CA) and cycling conditions described previously.[25] Electrophoresis of amplified products was performed using 1.5% agarose gels, with 20 5-mm-wide wells, run in 0.5× Tris-borate-EDTA buffer for 1.5 hours in a horizontal electrophoresis system at approximately 95 V. Gels were stained with ethidium bromide and visualized through ultraviolet transillumination with the Molecular Imager Gel Doc XR system and Quantity One software, version 4.4.1 (Bio-Rad, Hercules, CA).

Fig. 3 clearly shows a clonal outbreak of *S uberis* IMIs in this dairy farm with all isolates from the clinical cases belonging to the same *S uberis* clone. Based on the result of RAPD typing, it was concluded that this farm had a clonal outbreak of *S uberis* isolated from the clinical cases.

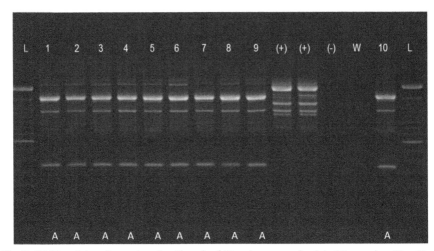

Fig. 3. RAPD gel showing a clonal outbreak of *Streptococcus uberis* in 10 cows in a New York dairy farm. Mastitis isolates of *S uberis* from the farm are in lanes 1 to 10. Lanes coded with (+), (−), and L are positive and negative controls and DNA ladder, respectively. W is a negative control lane with only water.

In this farm, data analysis, risk assessment, and infection profile all pointed toward a herd diagnosis of contagious transmission. The result of the data analysis, risk assessment, and molecular strain typing were reported back to the herd manager. Advice to resolve the issue focused on preventing infection transmission in the herd. Segregation of known infected cows was implemented, postmilking teat disinfection was changed to dipping rather than spraying, and milking equipment was upgraded to match the size of the milking parlor. Implementation of the advice was swift and clinical mastitis in the farm dropped dramatically over a period of 6 months to approximately 1.5% of cows per month.

Again, RAPD strain typing turned out to have a large value on top of classical culture-based diagnostics. Farm advice was based on the combination of data analysis, risk assessment, and advanced diagnostic methods.

Enterobacter spp

Enterobacter spp has been reported among the causes of clinical mastitis on dairy farms.[27] In general, no further speciation of the *Enterabacter* spp is performed. However, in several recent studies rpoB sequencing was performed and the dominant *Enterobacter* spp was reported to be *E cloacae*.[27,28] Clinical signs associated with *E cloacae* were generally mild compared with other coliform mastitis cases and spontaneous cure of infection is generally high. The authors report here on well-managed dairy farms of approximately 550 cows with a bulk milk somatic cell count of approximately 200,000 cells per milliliter. All cases of clinical mastitis were sampled by the owner and on-farm culture was performed. The owner noted a large number of gram-negative mastitis cases that were generally mild. Culture on the farm was inconclusive and further diagnostics were requested by the owner. Because the treatment routing on the farm was not to treat gram-negative mastitis cases, the identified cows with gram-negative mastitis remained in the lactating cow pen and affected cows were not segregated. The abnormal milk was discarded in a separate milking can, but no disinfection or elaborate cleaning of the milking unit was performed after milking the clinical cases. Data analysis on the farm revealed a relative high risk of new infections (~10%), with approximately 8% chronic high cell count cows. Risk assessment on the farm showed few weaknesses with excellent milking procedures and milking equipment that passed the ISO equipment test. The gram-negative isolates from the farm were tentatively identified as *Enterobacter* spp by classical microbiology. All *Enterobacter* isolates were subjected to *rpo*B sequencing and were identified as *E cloacae* (99% species identity based on 100% coverage of 900-bp fragment). All identified *Enterobacter* isolates were used for strain typing. Strain typing was performed by means of RAPD PCR.[6] Briefly, crude DNA extracts from *Enterobacter* isolates were obtained by 10-minute boil preparation and used as templates for RAPD PCR with primer set ERIC-2/ERIC-1026 (5'-AAGTAAGTGACTGGGGT-GAGCG-3' and 5'-TACATTCGAGGACCCCTAAGTG-3', respectively). Electrophoresis of amplified products was performed using 1.5% agarose gels, with 20 5-mm-wide wells, run in 0.5× Tris-borate-EDTA buffer for 1.5 hours in a horizontal electrophoresis system at approximately 95 V. Gels were stained with ethidium bromide and visualized through ultraviolet transillumination with the Molecular Imager Gel Doc XR system and Quantity One software, version 4.4.1 (Bio-Rad).

Results of strain typing are shown in **Fig. 4**. RAPD patterns for *E cloacae* isolates all showed a band of approximately 290 bp as shown in **Fig. 4**. Three different clones of *E cloacae* were identified: clone A was present in lanes 1, 7, 11, 13, and 16; clone B in lanes 2, 3, 4, 5, 6, 9, 10, 14, and 15; and clone C only in lane 8. Clearly, clonal transmission seems to play an important role in *E cloacae* infections in this herd, with two dominant strains present.

The results were discussed with the owner and it was advised to segregate all cows with clinical mastitis in a sick cow pen. After each milking of a clinically affected cow the unit should be disinfected before being used on the next cow. Cows will only be

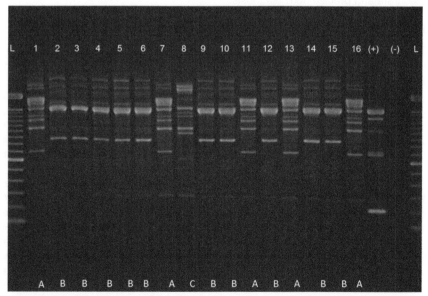

Fig. 4. RAPD gel showing a nonclonal outbreak of *Enterobacter* spp in cows in a New York dairy farm. Mastitis isolates of *Enterobacter* from the farm are in lanes 1 to 16. Lanes coded with (+), (−), and L are positive and negative controls and DNA ladder, respectively.

allowed to return to the milking pens with visibly normal milk and the absence of gram-negative bacteria from the milk.

Although *E cloacae* are generally not considered to be contagious organisms, the specific management practices on this farm with no treatment of affected cows and milking the affected cows within the lactating cow pens resulted in a high exposure of other cows in the same pen to this gram-negative organism. By eliminating this transmission route, it was possible to prevent further expansion of the clonal outbreaks.

SUMMARY

The use of molecular diagnostic tools has not changed the true pathobiology of mastitis or mastitis pathogens, but has definitely assisted in a much more accurate diagnosis and management of mastitis problems at the herd level. Molecular diagnostic techniques have contributed to the understanding of infection sources, transmission, and prognosis of major mastitis pathogens on a dairy farm. Using the molecular epidemiologic techniques, it has become possible to monitor spread of pathogens, to identify virulent strains, and to differentiate between environmental and contagious nature of infectious agents in the dairy farm environment.

In the coming years, with the advent of rapid DNA-based diagnostic technologies, the use of molecular diagnostics in mastitis diagnosis will become inevitable to improve the quality and precision of herd health management. The added costs must be considered, in connection with all of the technical benefits provided by the assay, when making decisions on implementation of the molecular diagnostic assays in routine mastitis testing programs. The authors have showed that genotypic methods are considered to be faster (in the case of RT-PCR) and more discriminatory (in the case of RADP typing) than phenotypic methods and therefore should be increasingly used in diagnostic laboratories. It has been shown that the combination of herd data analysis, herd risk assessment, and molecular diagnostic methods allows an accurate and precise herd diagnosis.

REFERENCES

1. Reyher KK, Dohoo IR. Diagnosing intramammary infections: evaluation of composite milk samples to detect intramammary infections. J Dairy Sci 2011; 94(7):3387–96. http://dx.doi.org/10.3168/jds.2010-3907.
2. Muellner P, Zadoks RN, Perez AM, et al. The integration of molecular tools into veterinary and spatial epidemiology. Spat Spatiotemporal Epidemiol 2011;2(3): 159–71. http://dx.doi.org/10.1016/j.sste.2011.07.005.
3. Zadoks RN, Middleton JR, McDougall S, et al. Molecular epidemiology of mastitis pathogens of dairy cattle and comparative relevance to humans. J Mammary Gland Biol Neoplasia 2011;16(4):357–72. http://dx.doi.org/10.1007/s10911-011-9236-y.
4. Levin BR, Lipsitch M, Bonhoeffer S. Population biology, evolution, and infectious disease: convergence and synthesis. Science 1999;283(5403):806–9.
5. Zadoks RN, Schukken YH. Use of molecular epidemiology in veterinary practice. Vet Clin North Am Food Anim Pract 2006;22(1):229–61. http://dx.doi.org/10.1016/j.cvfa.2005.11.005.
6. Munoz MA, Welcome FL, Schukken YH, et al. Molecular epidemiology of two *Klebsiella pneumoniae* mastitis outbreaks on a dairy farm in New York State. J Clin Microbiol 2007;45(12):3964–71. http://dx.doi.org/10.1128/JCM.00795-07.
7. Reinoso E, Bettera S, Frigerio C, et al. RAPD-PCR analysis of *Staphylococcus aureus* strains isolated from bovine and human hosts. Microbiol Res 2004; 159(3):245–55.

8. Struelens MJ, De Gheldre Y, Deplano A. Comparative and library epidemiological typing systems: outbreak investigations versus surveillance systems. Infect Control Hosp Epidemiol 1998;19(8):565–9.

9. Hata E, Katsuda K, Kobayashi H, et al. Characteristics and epidemiologic genotyping of Staphylococcus aureus isolates from bovine mastitic milk in Hokkaido, Japan. J Vet Med Sci 2006;68(2):165–70.

10. Aires-de-Sousa M, Parente CE, Vieira-da-Motta O, et al. Characterization of Staphylococcus aureus isolates from buffalo, bovine, ovine, and caprine milk samples collected in Rio de Janeiro state, Brazil. Appl Environ Microbiol 2007; 73(12):3845–9. http://dx.doi.org/10.1128/AEM.00019-07.

11. Tenover FC, Arbeit R, Archer G, et al. Comparison of traditional and molecular methods of typing isolates of Staphylococcus aureus. J Clin Microbiol 1994; 32(2):407–15.

12. Gillespie BE, Jayarao BM, Oliver SP. Identification of streptococcus species by randomly amplified polymorphic deoxyribonucleic acid fingerprinting. J Dairy Sci 1997;80(3):471–6. http://dx.doi.org/10.3168/jds.S0022-0302(97)75959-9.

13. Fitzgerald JR, Meaney WJ, Hartigan PJ, et al. Fine-structure molecular epidemiological analysis of Staphylococcus aureus recovered from cows. Epidemiol Infect 1997;119(2):261–9.

14. Nicholas RA. Bovine mycoplasmosis: silent and deadly. Vet Rec 2011;168(17): 459–62. http://dx.doi.org/10.1136/vr.d2468.

15. Justice-Allen A, Trujillo J, Goodell G, et al. Detection of multiple mycoplasma species in bulk tank milk samples using real-time PCR and conventional culture and comparison of test sensitivities. J Dairy Sci 2011;94(7):3411–9. http: //dx.doi.org/10.3168/jds.2010-3940.

16. Sachse K, Salam HS, Diller R, et al. Use of a novel real-time PCR technique to monitor and quantitate Mycoplasma bovis infection in cattle herds with mastitis and respiratory disease. Vet J 2010;186(3):299–303. http://dx.doi.org/10.1016/j.tvjl.2009. 10.008.

17. Jasper DE. Bovine mycoplasmal mastitis. Adv Vet Sci Comp Med 1981;25:121–57.

18. Boonyayatra S, Fox LK, Besser TE, et al. Effects of storage methods on the recovery of mycoplasma species from milk samples. Vet Microbiol 2010; 144(1–2):210–3. http://dx.doi.org/10.1016/j.vetmic.2009.12.014.

19. Rosengarten R, Yogev D. Variant colony surface antigenic phenotypes within mycoplasma strain populations: implications for species identification and strain standardization. J Clin Microbiol 1996;34(1):149–58.

20. Sachse K, Hotzel H. Classification of isolates by DNA-DNA hybridization. Methods Mol Biol 1998;104:189–95. http://dx.doi.org/10.1385/0-89603-525-5.

21. McAuliffe L, Ellis RJ, Lawes JR, et al. 16S rDNA PCR and denaturing gradient gel electrophoresis; a single generic test for detecting and differentiating mycoplasma species. J Med Microbiol 2005;54(Pt 8):731–9. http://dx.doi.org/10.1099/jmm. 0.46058-0.

22. Subramaniam S, Bergonier D, Poumarat F, et al. Species identification of Mycoplasma bovis and mycoplasma agalactiae based on the uvrC genes by PCR. Mol Cell Probes 1998;12(3):161–9. http://dx.doi.org/10.1006/mcpr.1998.0160.

23. Reinoso EB, Lasagno MC, Dieser SA, et al. Distribution of virulence-associated genes in Streptococcus uberis isolated from bovine mastitis. FEMS Microbiol Lett 2011;318(2):183–8. http://dx.doi.org/10.1111/j.1574-6968.2011.02258.x.

24. Green MJ, Green LE, Bradley AJ, et al. Prevalence and associations between bacterial isolates from dry mammary glands of dairy cows. Vet Rec 2005; 156(3):71–7.

25. Zadoks RN, Gillespie BE, Barkema HW, et al. Clinical, epidemiological and molecular characteristics of *Streptococcus uberis* infections in dairy herds. Epidemiol Infect 2003;130(2):335–49.
26. Zadoks RN, Allore HG, Barkema HW, et al. Analysis of an outbreak of *Streptococcus uberis* mastitis. J Dairy Sci 2001;84(3):590–9. http://dx.doi.org/10.3168/jds.S0022-0302(01)74512-2.
27. Schukken YH, Bennett GJ, Zurakowski MJ, et al. Randomized clinical trial to evaluate the efficacy of a 5-day ceftiofur hydrochloride intramammary treatment on nonsevere gram-negative clinical mastitis. J Dairy Sci 2011;94(12):6203–15. http://dx.doi.org/10.3168/jds.2011-4290.
28. Nam HM, Lim SK, Kang HM, et al. Prevalence and antimicrobial susceptibility of gram-negative bacteria isolated from bovine mastitis between 2003 and 2008 in Korea. J Dairy Sci 2009;92(5):2020–6. http://dx.doi.org/10.3168/jds.2008-1739.

Diagnostic Sampling and Gross Pathology of New World Camelids

Robert J. Bildfell, DVM, MSc[a],*, Christiane V. Löhr, Dr Med Vet, PhD[b],
Susan J. Tornquist, DVM, PhD[c]

KEYWORDS

- Alpaca • Llama • Camelid • Pathology • Disease • Diagnostics • Sampling

KEY POINTS

- New world camelids (NWC) may have up to 1.4% reticulocytes in circulation which makes differentiation of regenerative versus nonregenerative anemia difficult.
- Infection with Candidatus Mycoplasma haemolamae (formerly Eperythrozoon) can be associated with anemia and is best diagnosed by polymerase chain reaction assay using EDTA blood samples.
- Cerebrospinal fluid is a highly rewarding but underutilized diagnostic sample to work-up camelid central nervous system disease.
- Poor body condition due to dental attrition or malocclusion is common in older animals.
- Severe hepatic lipidosis may be associated with serofibrinous effusions and widespread petechia and ecchymoses.
- Cardiovascular anomalies are fairly common and can be easily missed unless the heart and large vessels are carefully examined in situ and in context of the lungs.
- Lymphoma is the one of most commonly diagnosed malignancies of NWC.

This article is intended to give practitioners an overview of diagnostic testing when submitting camelid-origin samples to a veterinary diagnostic laboratory (VDL). A review of some of the common gross findings and diseases when collecting these samples is included.

The basic principles for proper collection and handling of veterinary diagnostic samples have been reviewed elsewhere and generally apply to sampling of New World camelids (NWC).[1,2] Guidelines are often available online for each VDL and, when in

The authors have nothing to disclose.

[a] Department of Biomedical Sciences, Oregon State University College of Veterinary Medicine, 146 Magruder Hall, Corvallis, OR 97331, USA; [b] Department of Biomedical Sciences, Oregon State University College of Veterinary Medicine, 144 Magruder Hall, Corvallis, OR 97331, USA; [c] Department of Biomedical Sciences, Oregon State University College of Veterinary Medicine, 200 Magruder Hall, Corvallis, OR 97331, USA
* Corresponding author.
E-mail address: Rob.Bildfell@oregonstate.edu

Vet Clin Food Anim 28 (2012) 577–591
http://dx.doi.org/10.1016/j.cvfa.2012.07.001
0749-0720/12/$ – see front matter © 2012 Elsevier Inc. All rights reserved.

doubt, the laboratory should be contacted for specific instructions. The following notes regard some of the more common tests and the interpretation of gross observations in various organ systems of NWC.

HEMOLYMPHATIC SYSTEM

Unique anatomic features and common incidental gross findings include

- Spleen: white capsule similar to an equine spleen, roughly triangular shape and a serrated margin
- Lymph nodes small and sometimes difficult to locate
- Hemal nodes present
- Lamellated thrombus in splenic vein: blockage rarely complete, splenic parenchyma usually unremarkable.[3]

Notes on Diagnostic Testing

Blood cellular parameters of NWC are best assessed using EDTA samples and have been reviewed elsewhere.[4] Camelid erythrocytes are elliptical with a high hemoglobin concentration relative to other domestic animal species and some cells may contain diamond-shaped hemoglobin crystals (**Fig. 1**). Distinguishing regenerative versus nonregenerative anemia is difficult because clear criteria are lacking and nonanemic NWCs may have up to 1.4% reticulocytes in circulation. The normal camelid leukon is characterized by a neutrophil-to-lymphocyte ratio similar to dogs, cats, and horses, although the total white cell count tends to be high (8000–22,000 cells/µl). Platelets are small with azurophilic granules visible. The overall leukocytic responses to various insults or stimuli, as well as the gross character of bone marrow, are similar to those anticipated for other species. However, stress-induced leukocytosis and neutrophilia can be substantial, with white cell counts exceeding 40,000 cells/µl in some cases, including remarkable increases in band neutrophil counts.

Common Diseases and Gross Lesions

Subclinical infection with Candidatus *Mycoplasma haemolamae* (formerly *Eperythrozoon*) is common but can also be associated with anemia. Organisms can sometimes be visualized on blood smears as round or ring-shaped structures at the erythrocyte

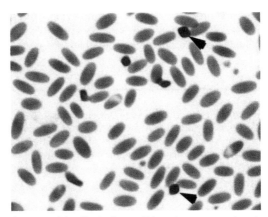

Fig. 1. Normal blood smear with elliptical camelid erythrocytes and rectangular hemoglobin crystals (*arrows*).

margin, but a more sensitive polymerase chain reaction assay uses an EDTA sample.[5] Juvenile llama immunodeficiency syndrome (JLIDS) is characterized by illthrift in young animals and can be diagnosed by flow cytometry methods using whole blood to confirm a B-cell deficit.[6] A more commonly requested test is assessment of plasma IgG levels in crias via radial immunodiffusion to check for adequate passive transfer of immunity as well as screen for JLIDS.

Lymphoma is the one of most commonly diagnosed malignancies of NWC in the authors' region and has been described by others.[7–9] The usual cytologic and histopathologic diagnostic procedures apply but it should be noted that, from both gross and microscopic aspects, lymphoma in NWC cannot be distinguished from a primitive round cell tumor neoplasm.[10] The latter entity is seen most often in younger alpacas and requires immunohistochemical (IHC) testing to separate it from lymphoma. This study found B-cell lymphomas are more common than those of T-cell origin are, especially if the gastrointestinal tract is affected. Diffuse enlargement of the liver (**Fig. 2**) and internal lymph nodes is common, but a variety of tissues can be affected.

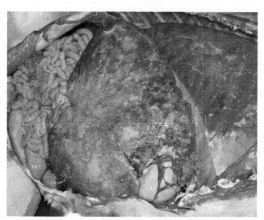

Fig. 2. Lymphoma in the liver of an adult camelid. The organ is swollen and diffusely infiltrated by neoplastic cells. A fibrinous peritonitis is also present.

INTEGUMENTARY SYSTEM

Unique anatomic features and common incidental gross findings include

- Microanatomy follows basic mammalian plan[11]
- Marked dermal thickening of cervical skin of intact males.

Notes on Diagnostic Testing

Identical to that applied to other species (eg, cultures, skin scrapings, biopsies). Serum zinc levels do not seem to be reliable for the diagnosis of zinc-responsive dermatosis.

Common Diseases and Gross Lesions

Review articles describe the breadth of conditions that may be encountered.[12,13] Hyperkeratosis is a feature of several of the most common entities, including chorioptic mange (**Fig. 3**). **Table 1** provides information on a few of the most common entities.

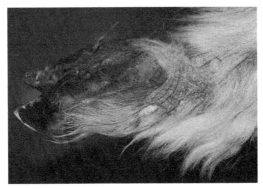

Fig. 3. Mild chorioptic mange on the foot of an adult llama. Alopecia and hyperkeratotic crusting are common features.

Table 1
Appearance and diagnosis of some common camelid skin conditions

Disease Condition	Lesion Character	Lesion Distribution	Diagnosis
Chorioptic mange	Crusting, scaling alopecia Variable pruritus	Perineum, medial thighs, feet	Skin scrapings
Zinc responsive dermatosis	Papular to plaques and crusts Nonpruritic	Thinly haired areas, especially face Often 1–2 y olds Dark-fleeced animals may be predisposed	Skin biopsy Response to long-term supplementation
Idiopathic nasal or perioral dermatosis (mange)	Alopecia and crusting Variable pruritus	Perinasal Perioral ± periocular	Skin biopsy Probably a reaction pattern to a variety of insults (eg, bacteria, ectoparasites)
Fibropapilloma	Raised, hyperkeratotic firm nodule	Facial May be multiple foci	Skin biopsy ± PCR for papillomavirus[42]

NERVOUS SYSTEM

Unique anatomic features and common incidental gross findings: none.

Notes on Diagnostic Testing

Cerebrospinal fluid is a highly rewarding, but underutilized, diagnostic sample during the work-up of camelid central nervous system (CNS) disease. Normal range for CSF nucleated cell counts in some laboratories is as low as 0 to 3 cells/μL with lymphocytes predominating over fewer mononuclear cells and rare neutrophils. Total protein levels may range from 31.2 to 66.8 mg/dL and glucose concentrations are about 40% of the serum levels.[4] This sample may also permit visualization of some agents or be used for specific immune-based reactions, such as serology or latex agglutination. At necropsy, the collection of appropriate fresh samples of CNS tissue can provide a definitive diagnosis for a variety of infectious agents. It is strongly recommended that half of the brain plus suspected areas of spinal cord damage be fixed in 10% neutral buffered formalin. Histopathology, plus or minus IHC tests, can implicate many agents, provide the diagnosis for conditions such as polioencephalomalacia and cerebrovascular accidents, or confirm spinal cord damage for conditions such as cervical spine trauma or spondylosis.

Disease of the peripheral nervous system seems to be uncommon in camelids, although histopathologic examination of nerves is sometimes rewarding, such as in cases of phrenic nerve neuropathy associated with diaphragmatic paralysis.[14]

Common Diseases and Gross Lesions

An excellent review of camelid neurologic diseases has been published by Whitehead and Bedenice.[15] Somewhat unique to camelids is the relatively high prevalence of cerebral edema, usually related to fluctuations in blood glucose or protein. A few of the infectious causes of CNS disease and best strategies to diagnose them are reiterated in **Table 2**. Occasionally, gross postmortem lesions, such as the cloudy meninges of bacterial meningitis, provide a diagnostic clue to the causes of CNS diseases but ancillary tests are typically required for confirmation.

Table 2
Diagnostic sampling for some common infectious diseases of the camelid nervous system

Disease Condition	Antemortem Diagnostics	Postmortem Diagnostics— Fresh Tissue	Postmortem Diagnostics— Fixed Tissue
Cerebrospinal nematodiasis (eg, *Parelaphostrongylus tenuis, Baylisascaris, Elaeophora*)	CSF – ↑ protein eosinophilia	None Rarely, adult *P tenuis* worms are found in the cerebral vascular sinuses	Histopathology
Equine herpesvirus I and arboviral encephalitis (ie, West Nile virus, eastern equine encephalitis)	CSF – ↑ protein lymphocytosis. Serum – serologic titers	Fresh tissue for virus isolation, PCR	Histopathology IHC
Listeriosis	CSF – ↑ protein, elevated cell count May see organisms Culture	Bacterial culture of hindbrain or spinal cord	Histopathology of hindbrain or spinal cord IHC
Cryptococcosis	As for listeriosis Also latex agglutination test on CSF and serum	Fungal culture May see malacic cortical areas grossly	Histopathology PCR
Bacterial meningitis (eg, *Streptococcus spp, E coli*)	CSF – ↑ protein, neutrophilia May see organisms Culture	Bacterial culture May see cloudy meninges	Histopathology

Abbreviations: CSF, cerebrospinal fluid; IHC, immunohistochemistry; PCR, polymerase chain reaction.

URINARY SYSTEM

Unique anatomic features and common incidental gross findings include

- Kidney unipyramidal similar to sheep and goats
- Renal pallor and swelling common in overconditioned camelids; corresponds to lipid storage in renal tubular epithelium.

Notes on Diagnostic Testing

As in other species, serum urea nitrogen and creatinine are useful indicators of renal function in NWC. Urinalysis is infrequently performed because camelid urine samples tend to be difficult to obtain.

Common Diseases and Gross Lesions

Congenital lesions of the urogenital tract are relatively common in camelids and can include various degrees of hypoplasia or aplasia, aberrant pathways for the ureters or urethra, and renal parenchymal cysts. Significant acquired gross renal lesions often reflect acute or chronic embolic bacterial disease, varying from large cortical infarcts to the firm, shrunken, pitted appearance of chronic interstitial glomerulonephritis. The authors have seen only a few cases of cystitis at necropsy, although urolithiasis with obstruction is occasionally diagnosed in male llamas.[16]

PERITONEUM AND PANCREAS

Unique anatomic features and common incidental gross findings: none.
  However, of note is

- Serous abdominal effusion with scant fibrin strands secondary to a wide array of disease processes, mostly related to hypoproteinemia and/or metabolic diseases.

Notes on Diagnostic Testing

Data published by Cebra and colleagues[17] suggest that parameters of abdominal fluid obtained by abdominocentesis include nucleated cell counts of less than 3000/µl and protein less than 2.5 g/dL normally; however, there may be healthy individuals with values outside this range. Identifying elevated amylase and lipase levels in peritoneal fluid versus that of serum is useful in the antemortem diagnosis of peripancreatic necrosis.[18]

Common Diseases and Gross Lesions

The gross appearance of peripancreatic necrosis at laparotomy or necropsy is a collection of chalky white foci of fat necrosis along the pancreatic margins.[18] A more common peritoneal gross finding is a fibrinosuppurative exudate, with or without plant material, usually reflecting either compromise of gastrointestinal wall integrity or sepsis. Often this fibrinous peritonitis is due to an ulcer located on distal aspect of the lesser curvature of gastric compartment (C) 3 (**Fig. 4**). A severe fibrinous peritonitis may also be seen as a component of septicemia due to *Streptococcus zooepidemicus* (alpaca fever).[19]

ALIMENTARY SYSTEM

Unique anatomic features and common incidental gross findings include

- Dentition[20]
- Gastric compartments; large C1, highly glandular C2, long tubular C3[20]
- Extensive spiral colon,[20] a common site for obstruction

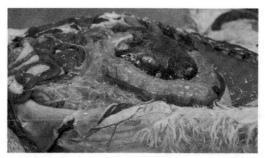

Fig. 4. Severe fibrinous peritionitis in an alpaca. This change was secondary to perforation of an ulcer in C3.

- Slightly pebbled appearance of esophageal mucosa (reflecting mucous glands)
- Gastroliths: hard green-brown concretions within glandular diverticula (saccules) of C1
- Lack of papillae on the mucosa of gastric compartments
- C3: minor cracks or fissures in normally thicker aborad third of C3 (acid-secreting portion)
- Proximal duodenum: ampulla and adjacent hair-pin turn are common sites for trichophytobezoars (obstructive, not incidental).

Notes on Diagnostic Testing

As for all species, a broad panel of ancillary tests (ie, bacteriology, virology, and parasitology) is required to adequately investigate infectious causes of weight loss or diarrhea in NWC. Fecal flotation using a double-centrifugation method with a sucrose solution is strongly recommended to detect dense oocysts, such as those of *Eimeria macusaniensis*, *Trichuris spp*, and *Nematodirus spp*.[21] During necropsies, the prompt fixation of histopathological samples from all levels of the gastrointestinal tract is recommended and these samples may be also used for IHC tests.

Common Diseases and Gross Lesions

Poor body condition due to dental attrition or malocclusion is often seen in older animals.[22] In the authors' region, enteric salmonellosis, paratuberculosis, and bovine virus diarrhea virus infections are rarely seen in NWC, but the approaches to diagnosis of these entities is the same as for bovine patients. Camelids may develop coccidiosis due to several *Eimeria* species but *E macusaniensis* deserves special mention because it can cause significant clinical disease in any age of camelid during the unusually long prepatent period or in association with low oocyst counts.[21] Some infections may become complicated by *Clostridium perfringens*.[23] Some features of common alimentary diseases are listed in **Table 3**.

HEPATIC SYSTEM

Unique anatomic features and common incidental gross findings include

- Liver on right side of abdomen, fimbriated appearance along the caudal edges
- Gall bladder absent
- Bile and pancreatic secretions enter duodenum via common opening
- Randomly located tan-white, 1 to 3 mm, mineralized granulomatous or fibrotic lesions, presumably sequelae to migrating parasitic larvae or episodes of bacteremia.

Table 3
Clinical features and diagnostic sampling for some common diseases of the camelid alimentary system

Disease	Clinical Features	Antemortem Diagnostics	Gross Lesions and Diagnostics
Clostridiosis *C perfringens*	Hemorrhagic diarrhea in juveniles	Anaerobic culture and toxin detection from feces	Bloody gut content Culture, toxin detection on fresh (<6 h) gut samples.
Coccidiosis *Eimeria macusaniensis*	Anorexia, lethargy, diarrhea, colic Hypoproteinemia Any age	Centrifugal fecal float with sugar solution for large oocysts[21] Fecal PCR[43]	Often normal but may see focal or segmental thickening of small intestine Histopathology from multiple sites
Coronavirus	Diarrhea Any age but especially juveniles	EM of feces	Fluid filled loops EM of content Histopathology and IHC
Cryptosporidiosis	Watery to yellow diarrhea in juveniles	Fecal sample, flotation Modified acid-fast stained direct smears IFAT, ELISA, PCR	Dilated large intestine Variable intestinal congestion Histopathology Fecal tests
Gastric ulcer	Anorexia Weight loss Anemia	Bile acids often found in C3 fluid[44] Abdominocentesis shows fibrinous peritonitis ± bacteria or ingesta in late stages of development	Often located in distal third of C3, lesser curvature Concurrent fibrinosuppurative peritonitis and hepatic lipidosis common
Giardiasis	Watery diarrhea in juveniles	Fecal sample—IFAT ELISA—only significant if large numbers	No distinctive gross lesions Test as per antemortem
Megaesophagus	Weight loss May present with obstruction	Contrast studies occasionally helpful Esophagitis rarely seen if scoped	Ring anomalies seen in a few young alpacas[36] Most cases are in adults and idiopathic[45]
Nematodiasis	Weight loss Hypoproteinemia Often anemia (can be severe with hemonchosis)	Centrifugal fecal float with sugar solution Lectin test to identify *Haemonchus*[46] Small numbers of *Trichuris* *Nematodirus* can be significant	Abdominal effusion Loss of muscle mass seen in most fatalities

Abbreviations: ELISA, Enzyme Linked Immunosorbent Assay; EM, electron microscopy; IFAT, indirect immunofluorescent antibody test; PCR, polymerase chain reaction.

Notes on Diagnostic Testing

Serum biochemical assays for camelid hepatic disease parallel those for large animal species with aspartate transaminase (AST) and sorbitol dehydrogenase (SDH) being particularly useful for hepatocellular damage, whereas gamma glutamyl transferase (GGT) best measures cholestasis. Bile acid levels can aid hepatic function assessment (normal range 1–23 μmol/L). Transabdominal hepatic biopsy can provide critical diagnostic information but, in rare instances of severe hepatic lipidosis, it has been associated with fatal hemorrhage (unpublished observation).

Common Diseases and Gross Lesions

The gross appearance of hepatic lipidosis in camelids mirrors this condition in other species; a pale swollen friable organ that often has a zonal pattern of cream and brown-red areas on closer examination. Cebra[24] has reviewed some of the underlying pathophysiology of this condition. Useful serum biochemical changes for this very common problem include elevations in AST, GGT, SDH, bile acids, nonesterified fatty acids, and beta-hydroxybutyrate. Severe hepatic lipidosis may be associated with serofibrinous effusions and widespread petechia and ecchymoses.

Fasciola hepatica can cause patent infections in camelids and the gross hepatic appearance of fascioliasis can include tortuous hemorrhagic tracks of acute necrosis, irregularly fissured areas of fibrosis, biliary tree accentuation with black parasitic hematin, and sometimes cyst formation with intraluminal thick brown exudate. Some camelids develop generalized cholangiolar proliferation and fibrosis as a consequence of apparently minor trematodiasis, resulting in a diffusely firm organ.[25] Another unusual sequel to fluke infection is fibrinosuppurative endocarditis.[26]

MUSCULOSKELETAL SYSTEM

Unique anatomic features and common incidental gross findings include

- Esophageal hiatus of diaphragm has cartilaginous ring.

Notes on Diagnostic Testing

Serum biochemistry for AST and creatine kinase are used for assessment of muscle health, recognizing the potential for a hepatic contribution to AST. Except for a slightly higher protein level, normal joint fluid parameters for arthrocentesis samples are not significantly different from those of horses.[27] Bacterial culture may yield various opportunistic pathogens in septic crias but septic arthritis is seldom documented in adult camelids at the authors' facility.

Common Diseases and Gross Lesions

Conformation problems, spondylosis, and degenerative arthropathies are common, but these seldom require sample submission to a VDL. The finding of serum hypophosphatemia in association with typical radiographic changes supports a diagnosis of rickets in young camelids, usually due to hypovitaminosis D, particularly in animals with dark-hair coats born during periods of short daylight.[28–30] Another common skeletal problem is swelling and distortion of the mandible. Although a few of these cases are neoplastic processes, most are the result of osteomyelitis, usually initiated by a tooth root abscess.[22] If radiographic findings are not diagnostic, aggressive sampling is required to penetrate the outer layer of reactive bone and obtain representative biopsy material plus samples for aerobic and anaerobic bacterial culture.

RESPIRATORY SYSTEM

Unique anatomic features and common incidental gross findings include

- Lungs: lobation and gross appearance similar to horse
- Nasal cavity: long and slender, obligate nasal breathers
- Edematous lungs develop rapidly postmortem, similar to small ruminants
- Alveolar histiocytosis: oval to linear white zones or clusters of small white foci along dorsal aspect of caudal lobes, not associated with textural change, correspond to clusters of alveoli filled by foamy macrophages (endogenous lipid) plus or minus mild alveolar emphysema.

Notes on Diagnostic Testing

Analysis of transtracheal aspirates has been infrequently reported. However, submission of wash fluid in EDTA for cytologic analysis, plus another serum tube aliquot for bacterial or fungal growth, may yield valuable diagnostic information.[31] Culture of samples of pneumonic lungs collected at necropsy is critical in achieving definitive diagnosis of respiratory pathogens, such as *Cryptococcus*, *Bordetella*, *Actinobacillus spp*, and *Streptococcus zooepidemicus*, and should be submitted in containers separate from samples of digestive tract. Fungi are difficult to recover from samples that have been frozen.

Common Diseases and Gross Lesions

Assessment of the respiratory tract of newborn crias must include checking for choanal atresia, especially if other craniofacial anomalies are present.[32] Crias with choanal atresia often have concurrent anomalies of the optic tract, brain, and/or cardiovascular system; a candidate gene for this complex of congenital defects has been identified.[33] A severe fibrinous pleuritis may be seen as a component of alpaca fever (streptococcal septicemia).[19] At the authors' facility, aspiration pneumonia is a more common diagnosis than primary respiratory disease in NWC and appropriate histopathology samples assist this diagnosis. Some cases are iatrogenic; others are secondary to megaesophagus or CNS diseases. In most cases of primary pneumonia, common pyogenic bacteria are isolated. Granulomatous pneumonia in NWC in some regions of the United States may be associated with potentially zoonotic fungal infections: cryptococcosis in the Northwest and coccidiomycosis in the Southwest, so appropriate precautions should be taken when collecting and shipping specimens.

CARDIOVASCULAR SYSTEM

Unique anatomic features and common incidental gross findings include

- Anatomy similar to other mammals
- Heart murmurs common in stressed animals may not have an anatomic basis, especially in older animals
- Arterial sclerosis with mineralization and even ossification in older animals; focal firm to gritty mural plaques in descending aorta and at branching points of large arteries; clinical significance unknown.

Notes on Diagnostic Testing

Cardiovascular anomalies are fairly common in North American NWC and can be easily missed unless the heart and large vessels are carefully examined in situ and in context of the lungs. When in doubt and when submission of the whole animal is not possible, submission of the entire, unfixed, and chilled pluck provides best results. Samples of heart for histopathology should include sections of ventricular septum and free wall, preferably including papillary muscle.

Common Diseases and Gross Lesions

NWC are prone to a wide array of congenital cardiac defects, including ventricular septal defects (most common); complex anomalies, including transpositions of the large vessels; and tetralogy of Fallot.[34,35] Vascular ring anomalies resulting in megaesophagus have also been described.[36] Endocarditis is not a common diagnosis but has been described especially in association with fascioliasis (see liver).[26] Endocarditis seems to be more commonly mural than valvular in NWC and vegetations may fill large portions of the ventricular lumen. Various septicemias, (especially *Streptococcus zooepidemicus*) can result in cardiovascular collapse with concurrent effusion of fibrinous exudates. Both antemortem and postmortem diagnosis of such conditions relies on appropriate culture of effusions or whole blood samples.

REPRODUCTIVE SYSTEM

Unique anatomic features and common incidental gross findings include

- Female tract similar to equine
- Male tract includes paired bulbourethral glands, a very small prostate, sigmoid flexure, and distally located cartilaginous penile process; lacks seminal vesicles
- Fourth membrane (epithelion) clings to fetus (**Fig. 5**); this delicate membrane is not the amnion
- Hippomanes (allantoic calculi) are often present in the allantoic sac
- Long umbilical cord occasionally results in abortion due to umbilical cord torsion
- Chorionic placenta is diffuse (no cotyledons) with minor variation in the density and/or length of villi (**Fig. 5**).

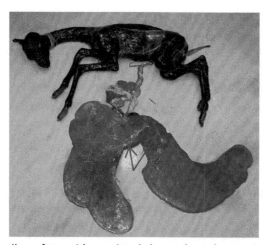

Fig. 5. Normal-term llama fetus with associated placental membranes. Poorly villous area on medial aspect of chorionic surface (*long arrow*). Amnion and umbilical cord (*short arrow*). Note that a fourth membrane (epithelion) also covers the fetus.

Notes on Diagnostic Testing

Diagnostic samples for infertility problems include uterine swabs and biopsies. The former are not useful unless guarded swabs are used because some of the common pathogenic isolates (*Escherichia coli*, *Streptococcus sp*, *Pseudomonas sp*, *Klebsiella sp*, *Actinomyces pyogenes*, and *Staphylococcus sp*) populate the lower portions of the tract.[37] Powers and colleagues[38] described a grading system for NWC endometrial biopsies that continues to be useful for diagnostic classification and prognosis.

Most cases of abortion or stillbirth of NWC are idiopathic and many of these are presumed to be stress-induced.[39] Placental insufficiency similar to that of equids may occur in NWC.[40] Therefore, it is critical to accurately determine fetal age (crown-rump measurements) and to collect multiple placental samples for histopathologic assessment. The pregnant (almost always left horn), nonpregnant horn, and the body should be sampled, taking care to avoid the medial aspect of the horns, which is normally villus-poor.[40] General principles apply in terms of collecting abortion samples and the panel of samples collected for NWC cases at the authors' laboratory for an abortion screen is listed below:

- Bacteriology—stomach content, liver, lung, and placenta
- Virology or molecular diagnostics—lung, thymus, kidney
- Serology—fetal thoracic fluid and maternal serum
- Analytic chemistry—liver for mineral analysis
- Histopathology—formalin fixed samples of placenta (multiple), lung, liver, heart, skeletal muscle, kidney, brain, and thyroid, plus or minus other tissues.

Common Diseases and Gross Lesions

Congenital reproductive tract lesions are common causes of infertility in both genders and may be confirmed at necropsy. The urinary tract or, in rare cases, the terminal digestive tract, may also be involved. Foci of placental pallor due to mineralization are common but their significance is uncertain. Abortion and stillbirth are common and often a cause cannot be identified.

ENDOCRINE SYSTEM

Unique anatomic features and common incidental gross findings include

- No unique anatomic features
- Thyroid glands of geriatrics may have incidental cysts filled with yellow to clear fluid.

Notes on Diagnostic Testing

Other than the assessment of reproductive hormones for pregnancy status and abnormalities in gonadal function,[41] antemortem diagnostics are rarely pursued in this system. Serum samples are typically adequate.

Common Diseases and Gross Lesions

Secondary effects of endocrine-related disease include hepatic lipidosis and the skeletal changes of rickets, but significant gross lesions affecting endocrine organs per se are rare.

SUMMARY

The general principles of diagnostic sampling apply well to the diseases of NWC. However, recognition of normal and incidental changes, combined with a focus on the more common diseases of these species, will maximize the return on diagnostic effort for these unique animals.

ACKNOWLEDGMENTS

The authors thank Chris Cebra and Pat Long for helpful comments on this article.

REFERENCES

1. Bildfell RJ. Collection and submission of laboratory samples. In: Kahn CM, editor. The Merck veterinary manual. 10th edition. Whitehouse Station (NJ): Merck & Co., Inc; 2010. p. 1463–9.
2. Webb DM. Getting the most from a veterinary diagnostic laboratory—a pathologists' perspective. Part II. Sampling and testing. Comp Cont Ed Vet 1995;17: 1043–71.
3. Hamir AN, Timm KI, Smith BB. Thrombosis of the splenic vein in llamas (*Lama glama*). Vet Rec 2000;146:226–8.
4. Tornquist S. Clinical pathology of llamas and alpacas. Vet Clin North Am Food Anim Pract 2009;25:311–22.
5. Tornquist SJ, Boeder LJ, Parker JE, et al. Use of a polymerase chain reaction assay to study the carrier state in infection with camelid *Mycoplasma haemolama*, formerly *Eperythrozoon spp.* infecting camelids [abstract]. Vet Clin Pathol 2002; 31:153–4.
6. Davis WC, Heirman LR, Hamilton MJ, et al. Flow cytometric analysis of an immunodeficiency disorder affecting juvenile llamas. Vet Immunol Immunopathol 2000; 74(1–2):103–20.
7. Cebra CK, Garry FB, Powers BE, et al. Lymphosarcoma in 10 New World Camelids. J Vet Intern Med 1995;9(6):381–5.
8. Shapiro JL, Watson P, McEwen B, et al. Highlights of camelid diagnoses from necropsy submissions to the Animal Health Laboratory, University of Guelph, from 1998 to 2004. Can Vet J 2005;46(4):317–8.
9. Valentine BA, Martin JM. Prevalence of neoplasia in llamas and alpacas (Oregon State University, 2001-2006). J Vet Diagn Invest 2007;19(2):202–4.
10. Martin JM, Valentine BA, Cebra CK, et al. Malignant round cell neoplasia in llamas and alpacas. Vet Pathol 2009;46:288–98.
11. Fleis RI, Scott DW. The microanatomy of healthy skin from alpacas (Vicugna pacos). J Vet Diagn Invest 2010;22(5):716–9.
12. Foster A, Jackson A, D'Alterio GL. Skin diseases of South American camelids. In Pract 2007;29:216–23. http://dx.doi.org/10.1136/inpract.29.4.216.
13. Scott DW, Vogel JW, Fleis RI, et al. Skin diseases in the alpaca (*Vicugna pacos*): a literature review and retrospective analysis of 68 cases (Cornell University 1997-2006). Vet Dermatol 2011;22(1):2–16.
14. Byers S, Barrington G, Nelson D, et al. Neurological causes of diaphragmatic paralysis in 11 alpacas (*Vicugna pacos*). J Vet Intern Med 2011;25(2):380–5. http://dx.doi.org/10.1111/j.1939-1676.2010.0661.x [Epub 2011 Jan 31].
15. Whitehead CE, Bedenice D. Neurologic diseases in llamas and alpacas. Vet Clin North Am Food Anim Pract 2009;25:385–405.
16. Smith JA. Noninfectious diseases, metabolic diseases, toxicities, and neoplastic diseases of South American camelids. Vet Clin North Am Food Anim Pract 1989; 5(1):101–43.
17. Cebra CK, Tornquist SJ, Reed SK. Collection and analysis of peritoneal fluid from healthy llamas and alpacas. J Am Vet Med Assoc 2008;232(9):1357–61.

18. Pearson EG, Snyder SP. Pancreatic necrosis in New World camelids: 11 cases (1990–1998). J Am Vet Med Assoc 2000;217(2):241–4.

19. Cebra CK, Heidel JR, Cebra ML, et al. Pathogenesis of *Streptococcus zooepide-micus* infection after intratracheal inoculation in llamas. Am J Vet Res 2000;61: 1525.

20. Fowler ME. Congenital/hereditary conditions. In: Fowler ME, editor. Medicine and surgery of South American camelids: llama, alpaca, vicuña, guanaco. 2nd edition. Ames (IA): Iowa State University Press; 1998. p. 468–97.

21. Cebra CK, Valentine BA, Schlipf JW, et al. *Eimeria macusaniensis* infection in 15 llamas and 34 alpacas. J Am Vet Med Assoc 2007;230:94–100.

22. Niehaus A. Dental disease in llamas and alpacas. Vet Clin North Am Food Anim Pract 2009;25(2):281–93.

23. Rosadio R, Londone P, Perez D, et al. *Eimeria macusaniensis* associated lesions in neonate alpacas dying from enterotoxemia. Vet Parasitol 2010;168:116–20.

24. Cebra CK. Disorders of carbohydrate or lipid metabolism in camelids. Vet Clin North Am Food Anim Pract 2009;25:339–52.

25. Hamir AN, Smith BB. Severe biliary hyperplasia associated with liver fluke infection in an adult alpaca. Vet Pathol 2002;39:592–4.

26. Firshman AM, Wunschmann A, Cebra CK, et al. Thrombotic endocarditis in 10 alpacas. J Vet Intern Med 2008;22:456–61.

27. Waguespack RS, Belknap EB, Spano JS, et al. Analysis of synovial fluid from clinically normal alpacas and llamas. Am J Vet Res 2002;63:576–8.

28. Van Saun RJ, Smith BB, Watrous BJ. Evaluation of vitamin D status of llamas and alpacas with hypophosphatemic rickets. J Am Vet Med Assoc 1996;209(6): 1128–33.

29. Van Saun RJ. Nutritional diseases of llamas and alpacas. Vet Clin North Am Food Anim Pract 2009;25(3):797–810.

30. Van Saun RJ. Nutritional diseases of South American camelids. Small Rumin Res 2006;61:153–64.

31. Gerros TC, Andreasen CB. Analysis of transtracheal aspirates and pleural fluid from clinically healthy llamas (*Lama glama*). Vet Clin Pathol 1999;28:29–32.

32. Whitehead CE. Management of neonatal llamas and alpacas. Vet Clin North Am Food Anim Pract 2009;25(2):353–66.

33. Reed KM, Bauer MM, Mendoza KM, et al. A candidate gene for choanal atresia in alpaca. Genome 2010;53(3):224–30.

34. Boon JA, Knight AP, Moore DH. Llama cardiology. Vet Clin North Am Food Anim Pract 1994;10(2):353–70.

35. Margiocco ML, Scansen BA, Bonagura JD. Camelid cardiology. Vet Clin North Am Food Anim Pract 2009;25(2):423–54.

36. McKenzie EC, Seguin B, Cebra CK, et al. Esophageal dysfunction in four alpaca crias and a llama cria with vascular ring anomalies. J Am Vet Med Assoc 2010; 237(3):311–6.

37. Tibary A, Fite C, Anousassi A, et al. Infectious causes of reproductive loss in camelids. Theriogenology 2006;66:633–47.

38. Powers BE, Johnson LW, Linton LB, et al. Endometrial biopsy technique and uterine pathologic findings in llamas. J Am Vet Med Assoc 1990;197(9):1157–62.

39. Löhr CV, Bildfell RJ, Heidel JR, et al. Retrospective study of camelid abortions in Oregon. Vet Pathol 2007;44:753.

40. Schaefer DL, Bildfell RJ, Long P, et al. Characterization of the microanatomy and histopathology of placentas from aborted, stillborn and normally delivered alpacas (*Lama pacos*) and llamas (*Lama glama*). Vet Pathol 2011;49(2):313–21.

41. Bravo PW. Reproductive endocrinology of llamas and alpacas. Vet Clin North Am Food Anim Pract 1994;10(2):265–79.
42. Schulman FY, Krafft AE, Janczewwski T, et al. Camelid cutaneous fibropapillomas: clinicopathologic findings and association with papillomavirus. Vet Pathol 2003;40:103–7.
43. Cebra CK, Stang BV, Smith CC. Development of a nested polymerase chain reaction assay for the detection of *Eimeria macusaniensis* in camelid feces. Am J Vet Res 2012;73:13–8.
44. Cebra CK, Tornquist SJ, Bildfell RJ, et al. Bile acids in gastric fluids from llamas and alpacas with and without stomach ulcers. J Vet Intern Med 2003;17:567–70.
45. Watrous BJ, Pearson EG, Smith BB, et al. Megaesophagus in 15 llamas: a retrospective study (1985-1993). J Vet Intern Med 1995;9(2):92–9.
46. Jurasek ME, Bishop-Stewart JK, Storey BE, et al. Modification and further evaluation of a fluorescein-labeled peanut agglutinin test for identification of *Haemonchus contortus* eggs. Vet Parasitol 2010;169(1–2):209–13 [Epub 2009 Dec 21].

Index

Note: Page numbers of article titles are in **boldface** type

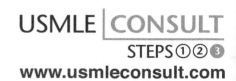

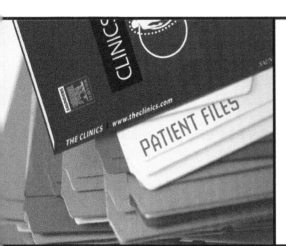

Moving?

Make sure your subscription moves with you!

To notify us of your new address, find your **Clinics Account Number** (located on your mailing label above your name), and contact customer service at:

Email: journalscustomerservice-usa@elsevier.com

800-654-2452 (subscribers in the U.S. & Canada)
314-447-8871 (subscribers outside of the U.S. & Canada)

Fax number: 314-447-8029

Elsevier Health Sciences Division
Subscription Customer Service
3251 Riverport Lane
Maryland Heights, MO 63043

*To ensure uninterrupted delivery of your subscription, please notify us at least 4 weeks in advance of move.

ELSEVIER

Printed and bound by CPI Group (UK) Ltd, Croydon, CR0 4YY

03/10/2024

01040439-0003